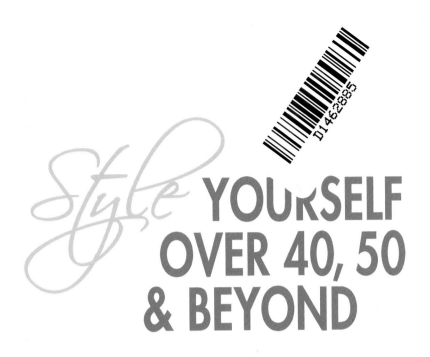

Style YOURSELF OVER 40, 50 & BEYOND

Create the "After" You're After!

SYBIL HENRY

The **Style**Concierge

Published by The Style Concierge, Marina Del Rey, CA
© 2011 by Sybil Henry
Printed in the United States of America

ISBN:
978-0-9839301-0-5 (Paperback)
978-0-9839301-1-2 (E-book)

Edited by Brenda Judy
www.publishersplanet.com

Cover and Interior Design by Carolyn Sheltraw
www.csheltraw.com

Front Cover Photograph of Sybil Henry taken by Shayne Nichols

Clothing and Accessory Drawings/Images by Juan Gutierrez

This book is printed on acid-free paper.

www.TheSyleConcierge.com

To all the women who may have feared their best is behind them.
Your best still lies ahead . . . you're just warming up.
Women over 40 get a second chance to be amazing all over again.
This is your time to shine!

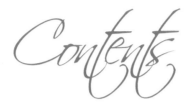

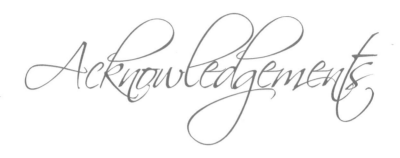

Acknowledgements

Many people say they have a book on their bucket list. I was no exception. I have always said, "I have a book in me," I just wasn't ready to begin writing until I felt I had something to say. Well, a funny thing happened on the way to life over 40 . . .

As with the accomplishment of any big bucket list item, it is not started or completed without the help of a few angels along the way. I did not have a shortage of them in my life during this process. They made this a better book and me a better person. I would like to call them out publicly to share my deepest gratitude and appreciation.

To Carolyn Sheltraw . . . Through your talent for book graphics, you brought my words to life and gave them style!

Many thanks to Brenda Judy . . . You gave me such a positive first-time book editing experience. From the day we met, I had complete trust in you. With your savvy perspective, eagle eye for grammar, depth of knowledge for flow and structure, solid judgment, and sincere honesty, you have shaped this book into something that makes me feel proud to share. You have taught me so much about writing and actually made editing fun!

Juan Gutierrez . . . I have no shortage of awe for the depth of talent in your multi-media skills. Your work is consistently incredible, with such speed and passion; you are truly gifted at what you do. I could not do any of this without you! I treasure you and the memories of our many collaborations. You keep raising the bar!

It is truly a gift to have a long-time friend who you trust, respect, and admire. Shelly Herrell . . . You are that special friend for me. Your brilliance and unique insights helped me early in this process more than you'll ever know. Your sharp feedback allowed me to gain clarity, maintain focus and stay the course. You are so kind and supportive; I cherish our friendship.

Finally, as with any large-scale project of passion, it is the family who bears and shares the brunt of long nights, sacrificed weekends and impromptu strategy sessions. This book would not exist without the encouragement and support from some of my most patient family members.

To my brother, Hilton . . . I have appreciated your positive feedback throughout this process; it has meant so much to me. Thank you!

To my sister, Dilva . . . As the professional writer in the family, it was a thrill for me to seek your advice on my budding writing career. Your keen sense of style and suggestions helped make me a better writer. I still have the writer's quote file of inspiration you gave me when I needed to take a break and get it all in perspective.

To my mother . . . Thank you for always encouraging me to follow my heart. I still have the "Follow Your Heart" pillow you gave me at the start of this project. Ever since then, I've taken the message to "heart." By having this constant reminder in my field of vision, I took it seriously and developed the courage to follow your wise advice. Thank you for all you do. I am eternally grateful.

To my daughter, Shayne . . . Oh, to be so young, talented and beautiful. Yes, as I always say, "God was showing off when he made you!" The artistry of your photographic eye has been a thrill for me to watch unfold. The depth and beauty of your written word continues to keep me in awe as the most captivated fan of your work. I will be eagerly waiting to see all that lies ahead for you. It has been more of a joy than you'll ever know to have shared this project with you and become your first client. You are the light of my life and a gift from God.

To my husband, Bryan . . . There are no words that could fully express, quantify or show the depth of my appreciation and love for you, but I will give it my best shot. I know what love is; it has been shown to me in you. Your unwavering expression of love—through your patience, encouragement, support and kindest of words—is the fuel that lights my fire. Your love has kept the flame of my desire burning strong for decades. You are the best example of what love is and I am fortunate to share my life with you. And, after all these years, I'm still hot for you!

Introduction

Congratulations on taking the first step towards making a commitment to a process that will take your style to an exciting new level!

You are about to begin a journey of self-discovery where you will gain insights and acquire new skills to enhance and transform your style. This book will become an invaluable resource to serve as a reference for all future style-related decision making. It will help clarify, maximize, find or reclaim your style over 40. It will help you style yourself over 40, 50 and beyond!

Arriving at the midpoint of life can be an exciting experience. You get an opportunity for a second chance to be better than you have at any other time in life. With experience and wisdom, women over 40 are truly extraordinary. It is during this time that many women find the strength and courage to do things they never thought possible in earlier years. While women blaze new trails in their lives and experience remarkable triumphs, it can also be a time for unwelcome and distressing changes . . . the size and shape of our aging bodies.

Hormonal changes lay the foundation for many sources of pain and shame about our body image. Usually beginning before or after the age of 40, we enter perimenopause—the stage of reproductive life before menopause when the production of eggs in the ovaries taper—and as a result, we begin to gradually produce less estrogen. In the last two years before menopause there is a sharp decline in estrogen. During this time, the body tries to adapt to the estrogen loss by finding other ways to replenish it. Fat cells can produce estrogen, so the body works harder to convert calories into fat to increase estrogen levels. As the body is trying to make this compensation, layers of fat are being stored in the body's "estrogen zone," located in the abdomen area. This is the reason women gain weight and add body fat, which changes our shape.

Whatever the degree of change you experience, whether it is mild or severe, it can alter your sense of confidence and how you feel about yourself. This is a time when many women change their style to camouflage areas of their bodies that make them feel self-conscious. This "hiding" can change the authentic expression of who they really are. Many women look longingly at a closet filled with clothing from earlier times when their waistlines were smaller or they weighed less. This reminder, sometimes daily, can lead to frustration and despair.

However, there was a time in our lives when we may have been comfortable with our bodies, enjoyed shopping and had more time for it. There were many clothing choices available that easily fit. We left the mall as excited as we started and came home with great new options to fill our closet. It seemed like, after turning 40, most stores and styles at the mall looked too young. We began our shopping trip feeling great, with the anticipation of finding something that would be "just right," only to leave feeling frustrated and discouraged. The music was too loud, sleeves too

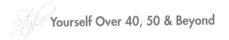

short, tops too tight, pants too low and, suddenly, we felt too old. Shopping wasn't fun anymore.

Many women over 40 want to look great but don't like to shop. The truth is that most stores in the malls cater to skinny 16 to 30 year olds, so it is no wonder that shopping may have lost its luster for some of us. In addition, with our changing bodies, we can't depend on garments to fit the way they used to . . . and that can be very frustrating! If this is how you feel, you are not alone; here are just a few comments from women over 40 expressing how they feel about shopping. How many of these thoughts resonate with you?

> *"I am afraid of losing my style, becoming old, irrelevant and out of touch. I fear that I may have peaked and my best days are behind me."*

> *"I want to maintain relevancy, maintain my appearance and stay attractive with sex appeal as I age. I still want to look hip but I hate to shop."*

> *"I am definitely over 40 with a body that is changing in directions that don't please me, and I need help to know how to dress it now."*

> *"Women over 40 are at the top of their game. We want hip, stylish and appropriate looks to show it; there are not enough resources for us."*

> *"I have been taking care of and looking after others all my life, and now it's time for me, but I don't know how to dress for my age and still look current."*

> *"I don't want to lose my looks, be out of style and become invisible."*

> *"I would like to age with some style and a certain current hipness."*

**It wasn't until I began my own journey of life over 40 —
as I experienced my own sources of pain
and challenges — that I understood the challenges
unique to women over 40.**

When I turned 40, I gained weight and began to fear aging. Once I became clear about how I wanted to age and who I wanted to be, everything changed—I lost the fear. I thought about what I didn't want and then created a vision for what I wanted.

I didn't want to morph into a frumpy old lady . . . I wanted to look modern and express myself authentically through my clothing . . . I wanted to be hip.

I didn't want to lose my quality of life. I wanted to be vibrant and energetic. I wanted to be healthy.

I didn't want to become invisible. I wanted to enjoy the pleasures of being a woman, feeling desire and being desired . . . I wanted to be sexy.

I knew I wanted to live hip, healthy and sexy over 40! I created a vision of who a hip, healthy and sexy woman is and how she lives her life. This became my map of how I would navigate myself through this time and become the woman I was meant to be.

A hip woman over 40 carries herself unapologetically and owns a style that is uniquely and authentically her own. Her style is a reflection of her essence on the inside that she brings forward to the outside. She is a savvy shopper and makes decisive clothing decisions that consistently reflect the clarity of her personal style and body shape. The unspoken communication of her style demonstrates to the world that she understands and accepts who she is, which radiates her personal power and confidence. She is well aware of the value she brings in her strengths and is lovingly accepting of her weaknesses.

A healthy woman over 40 is in charge of her body and is the biggest advocate for her own well-being. She is well educated about her body and the nutritional needs to keep her functioning at peak performance. She understands the value of regular exercise and has found activities she can enjoy that are compatible with her lifestyle and fitness goals. She measures and monitors her hormonal health—knowing it is the single most important contributing factor affecting her emotional and physical health. She knows it has more influence on her weight and shape than anything else she will eat or do. She has given up a lifetime of dieting, trading it for a new treaty that has an awareness and respect for her natural body rhythms based on self-guided intuitive principles rather than externally imposed rules and deprivation. She does not use food emotionally; she makes conscious choices about what she decides to put into her body. She faces her feelings, feels them, and expresses them assertively and appropriately rather than stuffing and eating them.

A sexy woman over 40 is comfortable in her own skin; she is self-loving and enjoys giving and receiving pleasure. She is no longer content pleasing her partner without it being a reciprocal experience. She understands that being sexy starts with her. She has taken responsibility for her feelings and starts by feeling sexy about herself. She is in tune with her body and knows her unique pleasure triggers. She communicates her needs for pleasure with her partner—knowing their shared pleasure satisfies and fulfills her. She enjoys emotionally healthy and fulfilling relationships with people who have shared values. Her environment is harmonious and in balance, reflecting her values and her lifestyle. Home is her source of strength; it is nurturing and serves as a place for renewal. She has made her bedroom a sacred space of sensuality, serving her deepest desires. She is interested in growing and stretching herself and is not content staying the same.

Once I clearly understood who I wanted to be, I started doing the things that would make it happen. I wanted to evolve into the person I was meant to be. When I released the fear, I was more open to receiving all that was waiting for me. I discovered aging is not about losing . . . it is about gaining. I learned it was my own fear mindset that was keeping me trapped—I wanted to move towards embracing these changes and finding solutions.

Through much trial and error, combined with my lifelong career in the apparel industry, I found a system that changed my life. It helped me gain a better understanding of my body, learn my authentic style and shop for my shape. I could visit my closet and find clothing that made me look and feel fabulous every day. This dramatically changed the way I felt about myself, how I walked out of the house and how I was perceived in the world. This change allowed me to accept aging in a more positive way.

The results of this process have been so powerful, insightful and life changing that I am compelled and committed to share them. There are so many women, just like me, who don't want to give up looking great in their 40s and beyond. This is not just a journey of fashion, but a story that is interconnected with fashion, body image and self-acceptance. I wanted to create a program that was accessible, easy to understand and had an interactive format. I used my experience from decades of helping others find and express their authentic style to become my first, best client, and then created this program for women to get their life-changing results, too.

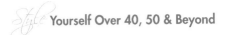

Wherever you are, you can be better. It's never too late to start. Some of you may be frustrated with your current state of hip, healthy or sexy. You may have lost your spirit or fear your best is behind you. You may not be as hip as you want to look, healthy as you want to feel or as sexy as you want to show. This can change. You can live the life of your dreams. No one achieves success alone, and I am here to help you with the hip part of your journey.

This program integrates the knowledge and insight from my diverse professional experiences, and my very personal journey—resulting in a unique perspective to help women over 40 look and feel amazing. I'll take you through a process that works from the inside out to help you gain clarity and pride about the way you look. Shopping will become enjoyable again, and getting dressed will become faster and easier each day. You can have a consistent, polished and personal style that you can count on. Life is so much better when you feel great and proud about the way you look. You feel lighter on your feet, have a better attitude and everything will feel easier to manage. We all know we are living our lives to the fullest potential when the beauty and power we know on the inside is reflected on the outside. This program is here to help you bring it out!

How to Use the Program

The book is separated into five parts. Each one takes you through sequential steps that logically build on the other. You will complete exercises that will help you gain important personal insights, which will allow you to reach your goals.

- Part 1 is focused on the inside to help you discover or recapture your authentic style.

- Part 2 helps you become an expert at understanding your body shape and how to strategically dress to keep your body in perfect balance.

- Part 3 gives you tools to plan, prepare, shop and assemble a balanced wardrobe that makes getting dressed a pleasure each day.

- Part 4 assesses your beauty maintenance needs—the defining details that make a big difference.

- Part 5 teaches you how to maintain your style for life.

Now, let's get started!

Sybil

Part 1:

IDENTIFY YOUR UNIQUE STYLE

Discover your style
from the inside out

To accurately and thoroughly uncover your unique characteristics, you will be following five sequential steps to uncover your style. We are starting from the inside out!

Step 1: Defining Where You Are and Where You Want to Go

Step 2: Assessing Your Style From the Inside Out

Step 3: Understanding How Others Perceive Your Style

Step 4: How Dressing in Your Authentic Style Makes an Irresistible Statement

Step 5: Find the Style Statement That Fits You

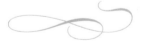

Step 1:

DEFINING WHERE YOU ARE AND WHERE YOU WANT TO GO

Setting a goal is the first and most important step towards beginning and completing the process of establishing your style. Your motivation to make a change in your style was so strong that it compelled you to buy this book; and this program will become an invaluable tool to help you make the changes you desire. While the goal of this program is for you to find and reclaim your style, there may be a very personal, individual goal that is unique to you. This personal goal often has a deep, underlying emotion that creates a strong motivation to propel you forward and complete the program.

Some of the changes women over 40 experience create deep, emotional feelings. We go through dramatic physical, hormonal and lifestyle transitional changes. These changes happen at different degrees of intensity—for some women slowly, and for others they even overlap! Despite the timing, these changes can prompt a desire to refocus attention back to you. Some of the reasons you may be inspired to focus on your style could include:

- Divorce
- Death of a spouse
- Dating
- Marriage
- Empty nest
- Financial windfall
- Career change or promotion
- Leaving the workforce or retiring
- Entering or re-entering the workforce
- Change in body shape or size
- Milestone birthday
- Neglected fashion, outdated wardrobe

Whatever the reason that motivated you to begin this program, creating a clearly defined personal goal will help you finish it. It is a well-known fact that goals are more likely to be reached when they are written. Once your goal is firmly established, the final step is to put it into action. There will be many opportunities for you to take exciting action steps in the later sections of this book. But for now, our focus is simply on establishing your goal.

First, give yourself permission to make your goal as big as you want it to be. Sometimes we are held back by old, negative thoughts from the past that limit our future potential. This is your dream . . . feel it, own it and take charge of it. By starting with a clearly defined

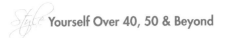

goal, you'll have a greater chance of turning your dream into a reality. If it feels too big at first, that's okay, you can step back, come back to it and read it again until you feel comfortable with it.

The goal you establish will become your guiding force, your North Star, lighting the path towards helping you stay focused and on track to complete this entire book. Your goal will serve as a powerful reminder of the reasons you wanted to make this change. Even during the most challenging distractions that may pull you in another direction, your written goal will be here to pull you back, reinvigorating you and inspiring you to stay the course.

So, let's begin with the basics. You'll start by completing a series of five questions that will set the tone for learning about your current situation versus where you would like to be. Make sure you set aside uninterrupted time to give this exercise your undivided attention; this is your foundational step. Take your time; if you don't have an answer for every question, just move on to the next one—you can come back to fill it in later.

1. How would you describe your current style?

_____

_____

_____

_____

_____

2. What specific changes do you want to make to your current style?

_____

_____

_____

_____

3. Why are you motivated to make these changes?

_____

_____

_____

_____

4. Once you have completed these changes, how will you feel about yourself and how will others respond to you differently?

_____

_____

_____

5. By what date do you want these changes completed?

_____

_____

_____

_____

Now, it is time for you to begin writing your goal. You can start by using your answers to the questions above and filling in the blanks below. Carefully review your answers. As you review them, determine which parts of your responses are the most compelling and emotion filled. When you identify your answers in this way, it will help you create the most personally meaningful goal that will inspire you every day. The goal structure format below will help you construct your final goal.

Your Goal Criteria Should:

- ✔ Be specific
- ✔ Be measurable
- ✔ Be a big enough change to be noticeable and excite you
- ✔ Have a deadline
- ✔ Include an emotional reason why you want it
- ✔ Be written positively
- ✔ Be no more than one goal
- ✔ Be short and simple enough to be recited by memory
- ✔ And, you should be able to vividly visualize it

Goal Criteria Examples

Be specific: I want to learn how to dress for my body and my age so I can feel proud about how I look

Be measurable:

I will complete all exercises in this book within in two months

Have a deadline: I will complete the program by September 1, 20XX

An emotional reason: I want to feel proud of how I look, end the drama of getting dressed, and be relaxed and confident when I go out on a date

Visual: I will find a photo of a beautifully dressed woman smiling while out on a date

Goal Structure Format

I specifically want to: _____

_____

_____

I will know I have reached my goal when: _____

_____

_____

When I reach my goal, it will be noticeable to me because:

_____

_____

_____

I will reach my goal by this date: _____

When I achieve my goal, I will feel: _____

_____

_____

This is how I will look when I reach my goal: _____

_____

_____

If I had to choose only one goal to accomplish, I would narrow it to this one: _____

_____

_____

Now, write your final goal on the lines below. Ideally, it should be narrowed to three lines and you may need to do a little editing to get it just right. It should be short enough for you to be able to recite easily from memory.

A Sample Goal: I will feel proud of how I look by September 1, 20XX; relaxed, confident and ready for a date.

My Goal: _____

_____

_____

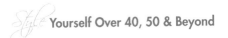

Excellent, you're on your way! To bring your goal into the sharpest focus, print it and place it in a visible but private location where you will see it every day (mine is by my bathroom sink). You may also want to place it in a small decorative frame to make it even more personal and special to you. The daily practice of reciting your goal will give you the greatest chance of reaching it.

The only way to ensure you track and monitor your progress is to make a commitment to your action plan. Think about the things you will need to do to make your goal a reality. You know what you want and when you want it; now, break your goal into mini steps, which will bring it into sharper focus and closer to reality. It is best to have at least three to five Action Steps that support reaching your goal.

For instance, in the Sample Goal, these would be the **ACTION STEPS** needed to make it happen:

- ❏ I will read this entire book within two weeks

- ❏ I will complete one exercise each week

- ❏ I will make a list of the supplies for my exercises, if needed

- ❏ I will shop for the supplies I need to complete the exercises

- ❏ I will put the steps in my calendar for the next two months

Your Action Steps:

1. _____

2. _____

3. _____

4. _____

5. _____

Step 2:

ASSESSING YOUR STYLE
FROM THE INSIDE OUT

Take a moment and, in your mind's eye, picture a conservative female teacher or boss you have had. Now, imagine her in the most conservative style possible. What is she wearing? Now, imagine putting her in the most outlandish, avant-garde outfit possible. Are you smiling? The visual of a conservative person in a wild outfit is repeated over and over in many sitcoms and movies. This image is funny because the outfit is such an obvious contrast to their personality.

While this image may be funny for comedic purposes, it is anything but when replicated in real life. This example illustrates how someone could be completely out of touch with their inner and outer selves. It is even more painful when it seems obvious to everyone else that they are not living their authentic style.

13

This is the reason why this book places so much emphasis on gaining insight into your identity and image. You get the most accurate and comprehensive view of yourself when your style is explored from the inside out.

To gain the strongest sense of your style, it is best to start from the inside with an understanding and acceptance of your identity. Your identity is the concept you have about yourself. The concept you have about yourself combines two major elements: your personality and your values.

PERSONALITY + VALUES = IDENTITY

Your **personality** is a set of traits you were born with and some traits you have learned. These traits are consistent and they make you unique.

Your **values** are the beliefs that are most important to you. These are the things you are unwilling to compromise. I like to refer to these as the "deal breakers."

When there is a consistency between your personality and values, your identity is very well defined. People have learned what they can expect from your behavior and how you will look.

However, when there is an inconsistency between your personality and values, there is confusion about your identity. This is the reason you will see style conflicts and it is how fashion faux pas happen. It is so important that you reflect upon your identity—it will give your style update the greatest amount of substance, consistency and authenticity. This reflection can begin by taking personality and value tests that help gain insight into your identity.

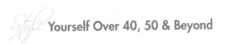

While this program does not attempt to put you "on the couch" and engage you in deep fashion psychotherapy, there are some helpful theories that can be borrowed from psychology. The "Five Factor Model," from *Personality in Adulthood* by Robert R. McCrae and Paul T. Costa, Jr., uses a well-known psychological personality theory. It is straightforward and can be very helpful in clarifying your style.

The following are two short questionnaires to help you begin the process. They will uncover some of the strongest aspects of your personality and values. Complete the questionnaires and, once you have finished, total your scores in each one of the five trait categories. This will give you an idea of which trait, or traits, best describe you.

Personality Questionnaire

Circle "Yes" or "No" and give yourself one point for each "Yes" answer.

Trait O

I have a rich vocabulary	Yes	No
I have a vivid imagination	Yes	No
I have excellent ideas	Yes	No
I spend time reflecting on things	Yes	No
I use difficult words	Yes	No
I easily understand abstract ideas	Yes	No

Total score   _____

Trait C

I am always prepared	Yes	No
I am exacting in my work	Yes	No
I follow a schedule	Yes	No
I get chores done right away	Yes	No
I like order	Yes	No
I pay attention to details	Yes	No

Total score _____

Trait E

I am the life of the party	Yes	No
I don't mind being the center of attention	Yes	No
I feel comfortable around people	Yes	No
I start conversations	Yes	No
I talk to a lot of different people at parties	Yes	No
I like to draw attention to myself	Yes	No

Total score _____

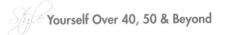

Trait A

I am interested in people	Yes	No
I feel others' emotions	Yes	No
I have a soft heart	Yes	No
I make people feel at ease	Yes	No
I sympathize with others' feelings	Yes	No
I take time out for others	Yes	No
Total score	_____	

Trait ES

I cope with stress very well	Yes	No
I remain calm in difficult situations	Yes	No
I often feel content	Yes	No
I am happy and enjoy my life	Yes	No
I am a peacemaker	Yes	No
My mood is stable	Yes	No
Total score	_____	

You have now identified your strongest and weakest traits. The two traits with the highest scores will give you a snapshot to clearly define your unique personality pattern. This exercise provides a foundation for you to understand your identity; but before it can be fully known, you'll need to clarify your values in the questionnaire below. Once you know your identity, it will lead you to eventually clarifying your Style Statement, which we'll discuss later in this section.

Values Questionnaire

Your values are the beliefs that you hold as important guiding principles for your behaviors and decision making. They are the beliefs that you are unwilling to compromise.

This exercise will help you better understand your most important beliefs. Review the list below and circle all the words that apply to best describe your values; then total your score for each.

Values – Trait O

Creativity	Freedom of Expression	Diversity
Freedom	Authenticity	Expression
Open-minded	Communication	Originality
Passion		Total: _____

Values – Trait C

Accountability	Efficiency	Precision
Appropriateness	Organized	Competency
Ambition	Sense of Urgency	Commitment
Reliability		Total: _____

Values – Trait E

Fun	Physical appearance	Glamour
Entertainment	People	Interaction
Femininity	Responsiveness	Sensuality
Connection		Total: _____

Values – Trait A

Helpfulness	The Golden Rule	Honesty
Simplicity	Community	Compromise
Nurturing	Friendliness	Family
Humbleness		Total:_____

Values – Trait ES

Endurance	Trustworthy	Routine
Responsibility	Balance	Quality
Consistency	Integrity	Dependability
Resilience		Total: _____

You have now clarified the traits that you value the most. With greater clarity about your values, you are ready to take the final step towards understanding all aspects of your identity.

What the "Big Five" Test Results Reveal About Your Personality

First, identify your **PERSONALITY TRAIT** (from the first questionnaire) with the highest score. This represents the strongest aspect of your personality. Then, find the name that matches the letter of your trait.

After you've identified your Personality Trait, compare the results against your highest score in the Values Questionnaire.

Trait O – Openness: Openness is a general appreciation for art, emotion, adventure, unusual ideas, imagination, curiosity and variety of experience. This trait distinguishes imaginative people from conventional people. People who are open to experience are intellectually curious, appreciative of art and sensitive to beauty. They tend to be more creative and more aware of their feelings. They are more likely to hold unconventional beliefs.

Trait C – Conscientiousness: Conscientiousness is a tendency to show self-discipline, act dutifully and aim for achievement. This trait shows a preference for planned rather than spontaneous behavior. It influences the way in which we control, regulate and direct our impulses. Conscientious individuals avoid trouble and achieve high levels of success through purposeful planning and persistence. They are also positively regarded by others as intelligent and reliable.

Trait E – Extraversion: Extraversion is characterized by positive emotions, the tendency to seek out stimulation and the company of others. This trait is marked by pronounced engagement with the external world. Extraverts enjoy being with people, and are often perceived as full of energy. They tend to be enthusiastic, action-oriented individuals who are likely to say "Yes!" or "Let's go!" to opportunities for excitement. In groups they like to talk, assert themselves and draw attention to themselves.

Trait A – Agreeableness: Agreeableness is a tendency to be compassionate and cooperative rather than suspicious and antagonistic towards others. This trait reflects individual differences in concern for social harmony. Agreeable individuals value getting along with others. They are generally considerate, friendly, generous, helpful and willing to compromise their interests with others. Agreeable people also have an optimistic view of human nature. They believe people are basically honest, decent and trustworthy.

Trait ES - Emotional Stability: Emotional Stability is the ability to experience and productively manage stress when faced with challenging situations and difficult emotions, such as anger, anxiety or depression. Those who score high in this area exude a sense of calm in tumultuous situations and feel generally content in life. Emotionally stable people value being rational and thoughtful, and their reliability and calmness tends to be reassuring to others.

Blending Values with Personality: Identity

Use the chart below to determine how your values and personality blend to form your identity. Write in your scores from both questionnaires, and record the total score in the final column.

Traits	Personality	Values	Total Score
Trait O – Openness			
Trait C – Conscientiousness			
Trait E – Extraversion			
Trait A – Agreeableness			
Trait ES – Emotional Stability			

The trait with the highest total score represents your **Primary Identity**—your strongest identity. The trait with the second highest total score is your **Secondary Identity**. Ideally, your highest score should be at least 2 to 3 points higher than your next highest score.

For instance, if your total score was 13 on the Extraversion trait, and your second highest total score was 8 for Conscientiousness, then Extraversion is your Primary Identity and Conscientiousness is your Secondary Identity. But, because there is a 5 point difference between these two traits, Extraversion is the dominant identity for you—you are not only consistently enthusiastic, outgoing and energetic, but you value these traits as well. It means that you are content with who you are and you value the traits that most define you. When your Primary Identity is this dominant, it means that your identity is very clear and defined.

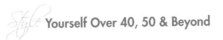

However, it doesn't always happen that your personality and values align so clearly. That means that sometimes the trait that received the highest score in the personality category did not get the highest score in the values category. The result is that there may be only a 1 or 2 point difference between your Primary Identity and your Secondary Identity. In this case, you may have a more diverse or eclectic identity. This can be a strength as long as you fully embrace these differences within your identity and find seamless ways to blend the different traits.

Hopefully, this second step in our progression towards identifying your unique style provided you with additional insight and clarity into your identity. This sharpened awareness will allow you to be clearer when you move towards understanding the next element of identifying your unique style: Your Image.

Step 3:

UNDERSTANDING
HOW OTHERS
PERCEIVE YOUR STYLE

Why is image so important? This is a question that you may genuinely ask, especially if you're a more internally focused person who thinks that being concerned with what others think could breed conceit, vanity or excessive focus on superficial qualities. However, to gain more control of your style and have it be an authentic expression of your inner self, a heightened awareness of your external self is crucial.

A willingness to focus on your image reflects your readiness to own your identity and present yourself to the world in a way that announces your personality and values unapologetically. When there is a full understanding of your image, and a consistency between your Identity and Image, you reinforce and promote the values that you most cherish. In addition, you are more likely to attract others into your life who appreciate the same values.

For some, this can be intimidating. When you authentically express your Identity in such a way that it yields a clearly definitive image, you are putting yourself "out there" for the whole world to see and judge. In my experience, it is the fear of judgment that often interferes with the development of a consistent and coherent image. Ideally, we should present ourselves authentically and unapologetically no matter who or what we are.

In an effort to understand your External Image, the following exercise will help you gain a better perspective about how you think you are perceived. It will give you a deeper understanding of how others perceive you, and you'll find out if your current Image is an accurate representation of your Identity.

Review the list of traits and qualities below and circle all that you think best represent the way others think about you. In doing this, reflect on things you've heard people say about you most often.

Image – A

Idealistic	Original	Distinctive
Independent	Unique	Creative
Refined	Imaginative	Unconventional
Modern		Total: _____

Image – B

Powerful	Conscientious	Quality
Appropriate	Goal-oriented	Professional
Strong	Dependable	Conservative
Credible		Total: _____

Image – C

Cheerful	Expressive	Provocative
Dynamic	Energetic	Bold
Gutsy	Dramatic	Open
Unrestrictive		Total: _____

Image – D

Warm	Unfussy	Casual
Affectionate	Informal	Approachable
Down-to-Earth	Comfortable	Unpretentious
Friendly		Total: _____

Image – E

Laid-Back	Loyal	Relaxed
Stable	Natural	Honest
Consistent	Calming	Authentic
Reliable		Total: _____

Add all the words you circled within each **Image** category and match them to the **Trait** categories below.

Image A = Openness: _____

Image B = Conscientiousness: _____

Image C = Extraversion: _____

Image D = Agreeableness: _____

Image E = Emotional Stability: _____

The trait with the highest number represents your perception of the **Primary Image** that you present to others. The trait with the second highest number represents your **Secondary Image**.

Now, from the Identity section, list your Primary and Secondary Identity (or identities if you had more than one primary and or secondary identity). Also list your Primary and Secondary Images so that you can compare them.

Primary Identity _____ **Primary Image** _____

Secondary Identity _____ **Secondary Image** _____

Ideally, there is a complete match between your Identity and Image. However, some variation could occur. It should not be surprising or troubling if the Identities and Images were reversed; your Primary Identity would be your Secondary Image and vice versa.

As with Identity, there could also be no Image that clearly emerges as prominently defining you. In such a case, it could be that you are a fairly eclectic person, and this is something that you appreciate and don't mind having reflected in your image. However, it could also suggest some ambivalence, image confusion or a lack of acceptance for some of your core personality traits. You could actually be wishing that you were different than who you really are.

There is only one real solution to this dilemma: you find a way to be more accepting of yourself. There is no bad personality trait; each trait has its strengths and purpose in the constellation of all human traits. Each of these traits is worthy of the fullest expression through your image and style, granting you the opportunity to live the fullest and most unique life possible. As you work towards and gain a greater degree of self-acceptance, it will become the most freeing and empowering experience for you. This acceptance will help you reclaim, or even claim, your unique style.

Now that you have a clear view of yourself from the inside, it is time for you to see how it is reflected and perceived on the outside. Our next step identifies and matches your Identity and Image with a Style Statement that represents you visually.

Step 4:

HOW DRESSING IN YOUR AUTHENTIC STYLE MAKES AN IRRESISTIBLE STATEMENT

Dressing in your authentic style is expressing who you are on the inside and showing it through apparel on the outside. It is a nonverbal way of saying, "I know who I am, I like who I am and I will be who I am." It celebrates accepting your shape, your identity, your image and the way you live.

When your identity matches your style, you project a consistent image that people come to expect. When your identity matches your image, you project a consistent authentic style that radiates confidence and creates a strong attraction. This is how you create your unique Style Statement.

When you connect your Identity with your Image:

- You appear "comfortable in your own skin"

- You gain trust from others

- You shop strategically and with clarity

- Your purchase decisions become purposeful and thoughtful

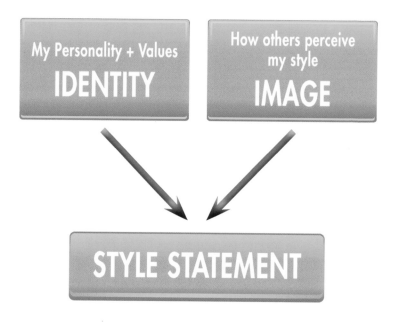

Celebrities have perfected Style Statement dressing. They are masterful at managing their image through style. For example, Oprah values people, education and communication. Her personality is warm, honest and dependable. She chooses soft, high-quality fabrics with mid-tone colors cut in modern shapes. She is always taste-

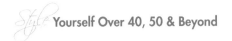

fully accessorized in small- to mid-scale jewelry. Her external image is integrated with her internal identity. Her image stays consistent with her identity, and she builds trust as an open, approachable, quality person with integrity.

Imagine if she decided to "change it up" and experiment with looks that took a radical departure from her internal identity. Picture Oprah in bold, eclectic clothing and flashy jewelry, something Sarah Jessica Parker might wear. It looks great on Sarah, but we would be confused if Oprah wore it. It would not be authentic or consistent with her personality, and she would lose credibility.

As we age past 40, we may need to rethink our image because, in addition to our bodies, our priorities and our self-perception may have changed too. A closet filled with clothing gathered from past years may have been just fine in our 20s and 30s—but after 40, they may not look or feel right anymore. It is not just about how the clothes fit your body, but how they fit your life and your style.

The first step in creating the style that defines you is "being true to who you are." This is important for your credibility and building trust with others. You know the feeling you get when you're wearing something that feels perfect, like it was made just for you. You feel good every time you put it on. It feels like "you," and you receive compliments every time you wear it. How would you like to have that feeling every time you get dressed? That is exactly where this program will lead you.

Descriptions of the six major Style Statements are listed below. They are a combination of your Internal Identity and your External Image, which creates an all-encompassing Style Statement. Review the following list, and find the style that matches your Identity and Image.

Openness   =   Chic

Conscientiousness   =   Classic

Extraversion   =   Glam

Agreeableness   =   Sporty

Emotional Stability =   Coastal or Global

My Style Statement is: _____

Now that you have identified your Style Statement, take a look at the brief descriptions for each. For your complete Style Statement profile, move forward to the page listed for Step 5.

The Chic Style (Page 39)

Your look is dramatic and creative, with powerfully confident looks dominated by clean lines and accessorized with one strong, unique focal point.

Values: Expressive, creative, communicative, free-spirited, passionate, unconventional, open-minded

Personality: Assertive, confident, competitive, dynamic

Image: Originality, creativity, independence, dramatic flair, sophistication

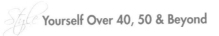

The Classic Style (Page 43)

You are always appropriate in simple, tailored styles with refined quality in timeless shapes.

Values: Ambitious, efficient, committed, precise, organized, reliable, competent

Personality: Intelligent, trustworthy, pragmatic

Image: Professionalism, strength, competency, practicality, conservatism, quality, credibility, urgency, dependability

The Coastal Style (Page 46)

Your style is refreshingly breezy; your laid-back style looks effortless in modern, comfortable shapes in calming colors.

Values: Open-minded, calm, informal, comfortable, flexible, patient

Personality: Relaxed and laid-back, unrestricted, open

Image: Simplicity, harmony, tranquility, composure, well-being, contentment

The Glam Style (Page 50)

All eyes are on you with your feminine, glamorous and body-conscious looks that are always perfectly accessorized.

Values: Fun, glamorous, interactive, sensual, people-focused, responsive

Personality: Charming, outgoing, cheerful

Image: Femininity, connection, exuberance, attention to details

The Global Style (Page 53)

Your clothing is highly personal, an extension of your compassionate nature and an expression of your values—you don't mind looking uniquely individualized.

Values: Nurturing, down-to-earth, fair, intelligent, conscientious, authentic

Personality: Empathic, humble, idealistic, optimistic, compassionate, wholesome

Image: Independence, integrity, commitment, originality, environmental consciousness, freedom of expression

The Sporty Style (Page 57)

Comfort rules—your look is approachable and energetic with a casual informality that always puts people at ease.

Values: Friendly, helpful, honest, family-oriented, humble, nurturing, affectionate

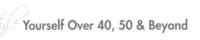

Personality: Warm, energetic, unpretentious, approachable, personable

Image: Athleticism, energy, practicality, simplicity, youthfulness, low maintenance

Move to Step 5 for a more comprehensive profile of your Style Statement.

Step 5:

FIND THE STYLE STATEMENT
THAT FITS YOU!

THE CHIC STYLE

Your look is dramatic and creative, with powerfully confident looks dominated by clean lines accessorized with one strong, unique focal point.

Trait: Openness

Identity: Expressive, creative, communicative, free-spirited, passionate, unconventional, open-minded

Image: Modern, distinctive, unique, imaginative, refined, polished, fashionable

Style Projects: Originality, creativity, independence, dramatic flair, sophistication

Shapes/Silhouettes: Clean structured lines, dramatic shapes

Styles: Tailored jackets with unique features through silhouette or design detail; long, shaped tops; sleek lean pants

Colors: Monochromatic with one strong focal point

Fabrics: Wovens and knits; you experiment with a variety of fabrics

Accessories: Large-scale, dramatic jewelry and scarves, or shoes that have unique designs, fabrics or colors

Grooming: Makeup is artfully and skillfully applied emphasizing best features, hair is sleek and fashion forward, enjoys variety in looks, always styled

Chic Style Icons: Halle Berry, Demi Moore, Teri Hatcher, Star Jones, Ann Curry, Courtney Cox, Jennifer Hudson, Iman, Sandra Bullock

Chic Brands and Stores: Michael Kors, BCBG, St. John, Donna Karan, Barney's, Banana Republic, Gucci, Zara, Chanel, Armani, Calvin Klein

Chic Fashion Magazines: *Elle, W, Bazaar*

Chic Style Profile: You are a fashion trend tracker who enjoys expressing creativity through clothing. You are most comfortable wearing styles with a dramatic, sophisticated flair. You prefer colors that are monochromatic to give you a modern, polished look. You also

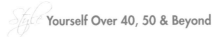
enjoy experimenting with new colors, fabrics, textures and prints. Your style says to the world, "I am open, creative and confident!"

YOUR CHIC STYLE VISUAL PROFILE

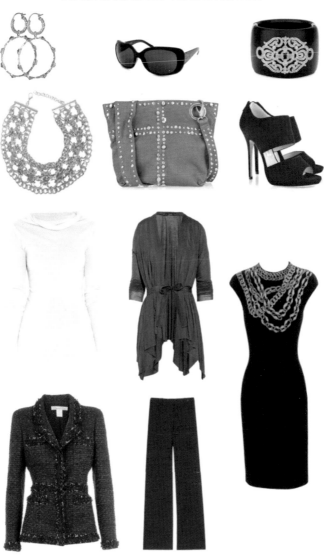

Chic Fabrics

Monochromatic tones with a variety of fabric blends and textures

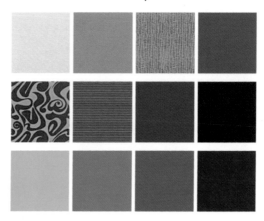

Chic Brands and Stores

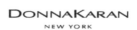

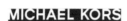

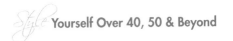

THE CLASSIC STYLE

You are always appropriate—wearing tailored styles with refined quality in timeless shapes.

Trait: Conscientiousness

Identity: Ambitious, efficient, committed, precise, organized, reliable, competent

Image: Professional, conservative, conscientious, powerful, appropriate

Style Projects: Professionalism, strength, competency, practicality, conservatism, quality, credibility, urgency, dependability

Shapes/Silhouettes: Traditional lines, clean and unfussy

Styles: Tailored jackets, crisp collared shirts, matching or coordinated cardigan sets, wears pants at natural waist

Colors: You prefer solid colors and are most comfortable in earth tones

Fabrics: Crisp woven fabrics, natural fibers, traditional patterns and solids

Accessories: Small- to medium-scale jewelry; high-quality pieces; low to moderate heel shoes, often matching the color of your outfit

Grooming: Soft and natural looking makeup, hair is simple and neat in one length or a few layers

Classic Style Icons: Barbra Walters, Jane Fonda, Michelle Obama, Martha Stewart, Clare Dane, Oprah, Hillary Swank, Cate Blanchett, Gwyneth Paltrow, Kate Winslet, Nicole Kidman

Classic Brands and Stores: Ann Klein, Coach, Dockers, Doncaster, Ellen Tracy, Izod, Jones New York, Liz Claiborne, Coach, Ralph Lauren, Ann Taylor, Brooks Brothers, Burberry, Faconnable, Talbots, Classiques Entier

Classic Magazines: *More, Vogue, Ladies Home Journal*

Classic Style Profile: You are traditional with a modern interpretation. You are most comfortable wearing tailored styles in crisp fabrics. You prefer solid color neutral shades with a bright pop and a few small-scale patterns. Your style says to the world, "You can count on me."

YOUR CLASSIC STYLE VISUAL PROFILE

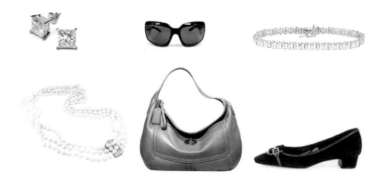

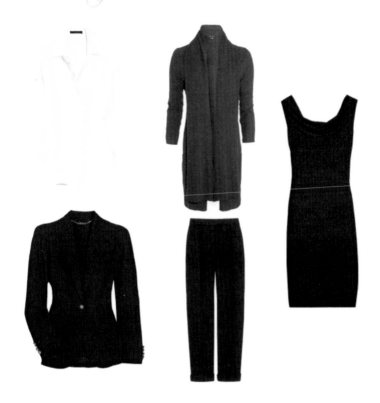

Classic Fabrics

Crisp woven natural fibers in earth tones, traditional patterns and solids

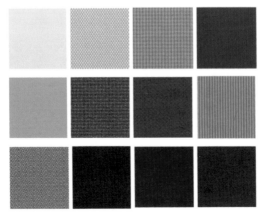

Classic Brands and Stores

  BANANA REPUBLIC

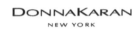

GUCCI

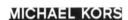

THE COASTAL STYLE

Your style is refreshingly breezy with laid-back ease in modern, comfortable shapes and calming colors.

Trait: Emotional Stability

Identity: Open-minded, calm, informal, comfortable, flexible, patient

Image: Relaxed, laid-back, unrestricted, open, effortless, mellow

Style Projects: Simplicity, harmony, tranquility, composure, well-being, contentment

Shapes/Silhouettes: Laid-back looks in lean or relaxed shapes

Styles: Casual and sophisticated, sleeveless tanks and tops, breezy tunics over relaxed pants, and open-toe shoes

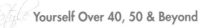

Colors: Sun-drenched brights, mid-tone solids and a touch of sea-inspired prints

Fabrics: Soft, comfortable knits, natural woven fabrics and a few pieces of denim

Accessories: Simple accessories, silver jewelry, always sunglasses

Grooming: Makeup is natural and easy with a sun-kissed low maintenance style. Hair is loose and casual.

Coastal Style Icons: Christie Brinkley, Jennifer Anniston, Cindy Crawford

Coastal Brands: Lilly Pulitzer, Newport News, J. Jill

Coastal Stores: Tommy Bahama, Coldwater Creek, Chico's

Coastal Magazines: *Coastal Living*

Coastal Style Profile: Your style has casual sophistication with laid-back ease. You are most comfortable wearing styles in simple shapes and natural fabrics. You prefer solid colors in vibrant or sun-washed shades, nautical stripes or tropical inspired patterns. Your style says to the world, "Every day is like a vacation."

YOUR COASTAL STYLE VISUAL PROFILE

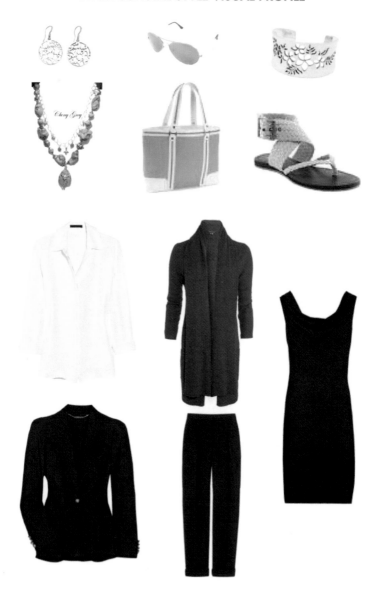

Coastal Fabrics

Mid-tone solids, sun-drenched brights, a touch of sea-inspired prints and denim accents

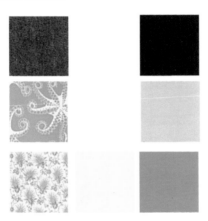

Coastal Brands and Stores

chico's   *Coldwater Creek*   J.Jill

    NEWPORT NEWS

Lilly   Garnet Hill   Tommy Bahama
original designs in clothing and home decor

THE GLAM STYLE

All eyes are on you with your feminine, glamorous and body-conscious looks that are always perfectly accessorized.

Trait: Extraversion

Identity: Fun, glamorous, interactive, sensual, people-focused, responsive

Image: Cheerful, energetic, expressive, bold, provocative, uninhibited

Style Projects: Femininity, connection, exuberance, attention to details

Shapes/Silhouettes: Close fitting, body-conscious clothing

Styles: An emphasis on showing the shape of the body with low-cut feminine tops, form-fitting pants, slim skirts, wrap and sweater dresses

Colors: Bold, graphic high-contrast colors, enjoys wearing animal prints

Fabrics: Shiny, fluffy, stretchy, soft, sensual fabrics that feel good against the skin

Accessories: Jewelry is abundant and bold; often wears high heels

Grooming: Medium to long hair worn with volume through layering, curls or waves; experiments with coloring. Enjoys makeup and emphasizes eyes and lips.

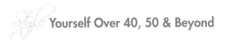

Glam Style Icons: Jennifer Lopez, Salma Hayek, Catherine Zeta-Jones, Vanessa Williams, Mary J. Blige, Sofia Verega, Mariah Carey

Glam Stores and Brands: Baby Phat, Diane Von Furstenburg, Dolce and Gabbana, Guess, Rock and Republic, Arden B., Bebe, Cache, Victoria's Secret, Juicy Couture

Glam Magazines: *In Style*

Glam Style Profile: You are glamorous and enjoy connecting with others. You are most comfortable wearing styles that are feminine to show your shape. You prefer colors that stand out in a crowd and make a statement. Your style says to the world, "I enjoy expressing myself and won't shy away from attention!"

YOUR GLAM STYLE VISUAL PROFILE

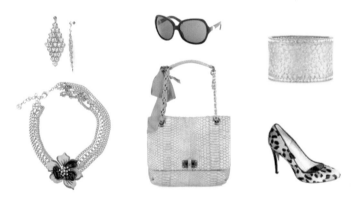

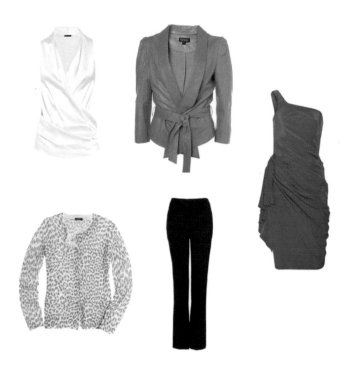

Glam Fabrics

Soft, sensual fabrics that feel good against the skin with feminine, glamorous appeal

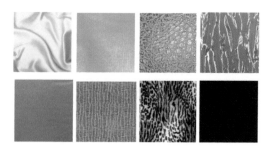

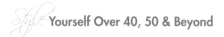

Glam Brands and Stores

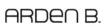

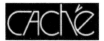

THE GLOBAL STYLE

Your clothing is highly personal, an extension of your compassionate nature and an expression of your values—you don't mind looking uniquely individualized.

Trait: Emotional Stability

Identity: Nurturing, down-to-earth, fair, intelligent, conscientious, authentic

Image: Empathic, humble, idealistic, optimistic, compassionate, wholesome

Style Projects: Independence, integrity, commitment, originality, environmental consciousness, freedom of expression

Shapes/Silhouettes: Loose, long and layered

Style: Relaxed and funky styles, ethnic or vintage inspired; unique, flowing shapes in colorful prints.

Colors: Rich, warm colors with earth tones serve as a foundation to the palette with vibrant accents

Fabrics: Natural, soft fabrics that drape and layer well

Accessories: Artistic or artisan accessories, unconventional designs that allow for personal expression

Grooming: Hair and makeup are natural and modern

Global Style Icons: Sheryl Crow, Goldie Hawn, Diane Keaton, Sarah Jessica Parker, Lisa Bonet, Susan Sarandon, Gwen Stefani

Global Stores and Brands: Anthropologie, Betsy Johnson, Eileen Fisher, Trina Turk, Tory Burch, Lucky Brand

Global Fashion Magazines: *O*, *Real Simple*

Global Style Profile: You are most comfortable wearing styles that have an individual expression. You prefer punctuating outfits with unique accessories that project your personal values. Your style says to the world, "I stay true to myself and follow my own lead."

YOUR GLOBAL STYLE VISUAL PROFILE

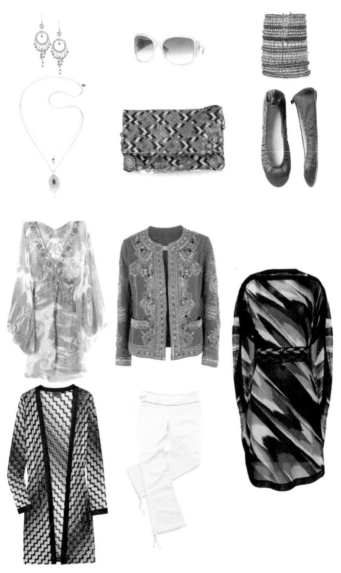

Global Fabrics

Rich, warm earth tones serve as a foundation to the palette with vibrant print accents

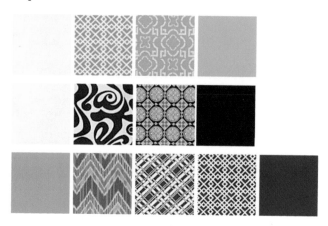

Global Brands and Stores

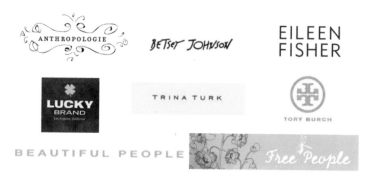

THE SPORTY STYLE

Comfort rules—your look is approachable and energetic with a casual informality that always puts people at ease.

Trait: Agreeableness

Identity: Friendly, helpful, honest, family-oriented, humble, nurturing, affectionate

Image: Warm, unpretentious, approachable, casual, comfortable, informal. outdoorsy

Style Projects: Athleticism, energy, practicality, simplicity, youthfulness, low maintenance

Shapes/Silhouettes: Unconstructed, functional, sports-inspired simple shapes

Styles: Casual jackets, T-shirts, jeans, shorts

Colors: Solid earth tones contrasted with bright primary colors

Fabrics: Easy-care fabrics in natural and technical blends for breathable comfort, stretch knits for ease of movement, denim

Accessories: Practical and small-scale jewelry, low-heel soft shoes, especially tennis shoes

Grooming: Makeup is clean and natural looking. Hair is unfussy, neat and natural

Sporty Style Icons: Whoopi Goldberg, Meg Ryan, Ellen DeGeneris, Jennifer Garner, Carmen Diaz

Sporty Brands and Stores: DKNY, Jones NY Sport, Lacoste, Land's End, Levis, Gap, L.L. Bean, The North Face, Old Navy, Patagonia, REI, Ann Taylor Loft

Sporty Magazines: *Shape, Fitness*

Sporty Style Profile: You are open, friendly and approachable. You are at ease in simple styles that are uncomplicated and efficient, allowing freedom of movement. You prefer wearing earth tone colors with bright contrasting accents. Your style says to the world, "I am comfortable!"

YOUR SPORTY STYLE VISUAL PROFILE

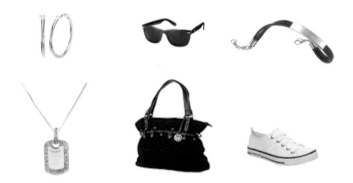

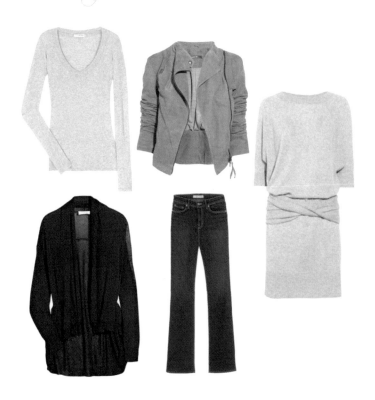

Sporty Fabric Profile

Solid earth tones contrasted with bright primary colors and denim

Sporty Brands and Stores

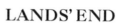

LANDS' END L.L.Bean

OLD NAVY patagonia

Part 2:

DRESS FOR YOUR SHAPE

Become an expert at
understanding your body

Being comfortable with your body allows you to fully express your authentic style over 40. But to feel comfortable and look great, it is important for you to be the best expert about your own body. When you clearly understand your body proportions, how they relate in relation to other body parts, and how to accentuate or camouflage your shape, you will be an expert!

Step 1: Understanding Your Horizontal Body

Step 2: Clothing Strategies to Balance Your Horizontal Body

Step 3: Understanding Your Vertical Body

Step 4: Clothing Strategies to Balance Your Vertical Body

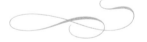

Step 1:

UNDERSTANDING YOUR HORIZONTAL BODY

It is rare for a woman's body to be in perfect symmetrical balance. As we age, symmetry becomes even more difficult—making it ever more important that you understand your body, your proportions, and how to dress strategically. Through simple techniques, you can artfully manage body changes with fashion strategies that give the illusion of perfect balance and harmonious symmetry.

Our eye is naturally drawn to balance and symmetry; in fashion, a balanced body suggests the look of vitality, youth and beauty. There are two main shape characteristics that define your body type. They are your **horizontal** and **vertical** measurements.

But first, it is important to know which horizontal and vertical measurements are in balance and which ones are out of balance before learning how to adjust them.

We'll start with your horizontal measurements. Most women are familiar with the "fruit and angle" term so, for the sake of fast and easy reference, I'll be using this terminology.

Five main descriptive shapes define the **Horizontal Body Proportion**:

1. Pear
2. Hourglass
3. Apple
4. Rectangle
5. Inverted Triangle

By taking measurements across your shoulders, waist and hips, it will identify your horizontal body shape. The information you gather from taking these measurements will guide you towards knowing which one of the five horizontal shapes describe you the best. Once you know your body shape, you will be able to easily choose styles and accessories that create a perfectly balanced body.

There are several ways to determine your horizontal body shape, but I prefer to use the following method because it is so easy to understand and is accurate. It takes into account the horizontal lines of your body that extend out the farthest—the angles our eyes see first. These are the most extreme lines of your body and they create your horizontal shape. The widest lines are your shoulders and hips—the narrowest is your waist.

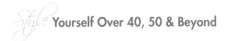

How to measure:

You'll need a full or 3/4-length mirror and a measuring tape.

Dress in underwear or, if you prefer, you can be naked.

Stand straight in front of the mirror with the tape measure and take "flat" measurements (do not measure the circumference of your body, just straight across the front of your body from one end point to the other).

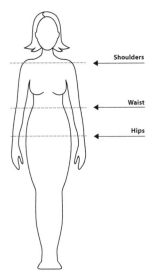

Shoulders: Measure in a flat, straight line from the end of one shoulder to the end of the other shoulder.

Waist: Find the narrowest part of your torso to locate your waist (you can bend to the side to see where it indents) and measure it in a flat, straight line, from one side to the other.

Hips: Find the widest part of your hips—measure in a flat, straight line from one end to the other.

My flat shoulder measurement is: _____

My flat waist measurement is: _____

My flat hip measurement is: _____

Now that you have your three horizontal measurements, review the chart below to find the shape that matches your measurements.

Pear

You have a pear shape if your shoulders are smaller than your hips.

Hourglass

You have an hourglass shape if your shoulders and hip measurements are the same and your waist is at least 2 to 3 inches smaller.

Apple

You have an apple shape if your waist measurement is larger than your shoulders and hips.

Rectangle

You have a rectangle shape if your shoulders, waist and hip measurements are the same.

Inverted Triangle

You have an inverted triangle shape if your shoulders are larger than your hips.

My horizontal body shape is _____

$\mathscr{Step}$ 2:

CLOTHING STRATEGIES TO BALANCE YOUR HORIZONTAL BODY

Now that you have identified the shape of your horizontal body, we'll discuss the clothing strategies that will help you achieve the look of "perfect balance"!

Every woman is beautiful. Despite the media images we see every day that attempt to give us messages that we are not good enough until we buy their product or wear their garment, we are more than good enough. This daily barrage over a lifetime can wear down even the most confident woman and affect her body image.

But first, I'd like to take a moment to talk about the perceived body imperfections that cause so much self-loathing and grief for women. Sometimes we can lose sight of all that is beautiful in the face of the areas we dislike. While the truth is that it is rare for the body to have perfect proportion, it can also be true that our perfection lies in our imperfections.

Every woman is beautiful in her own way. While it may be a stretch to ask you to love your entire body, there are spectacular parts for you to claim as beautiful. In an effort to bring a balanced perspective of your body, I would like to highlight the beautiful parts.

One of the best strategies to use when making clothing decisions and planning outfits is to accentuate your best asset. I call this working with your **Zone of Beauty.** Your Zone of Beauty is the most beautiful part of, or area of, your body.

When you identify and claim your Zone of Beauty, it will further empower and elevate your style. In addition, it:

- Becomes the focal point for your style
- Helps you identify and claim the most beautiful parts of your body
- Creates a higher level of awareness and appreciation of your body
- Gives you a boost of confidence for a more positive body image

While the reality is that no body is in perfect proportion, when working to achieve balance, there will be attention brought to the areas that are out of balance. As a result, this may feel discouraging and provoke negative body thoughts. Our goal is to highlight and accentuate the positives while camouflaging the areas that are out of balance. While doing this, it will be important not to lose sight of how powerful the beautiful areas will be and that they will draw far more attention than the areas that will be de-emphasized.

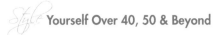

Each body shape has a specific Zone of Beauty to bring forward and embellish. Find your shape and advance to that page to learn more about your most special Zone(s) and clothing strategies that will help you achieve a look of perfect balance.

Pear – **Page 69**   Hourglass – **Page 72**   Apple – **Page 74**
Rectangle – **Page 77**   Inverted Triangle – **Page 80**

PEAR

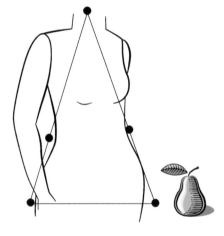

The width of your shoulders is smaller than your hips.

Zone of Beauty: Waistline or Hips

The pear shape is the most eye-catching, man pleasing body type of them all! Many pear-shaped women confide in me that they feel self-conscious or embarrassed about their hips, thighs and butts. They think they are too big, or even fat, because of the extra weight in the lower half of their bodies. Well ladies, I am here to tell you that from a man's perspective (they've confided in me, too), they can't get enough of an eyeful of your "curvelicious" body—no matter what your size, it's your shape that they love. In addition, the women of other body shapes dream about having the shape and size of your beautiful, bountiful backside.

Your smaller upper body gives you an exaggeration of a curvy frame in contrast to your fuller lower body. Make the most of it by bringing focus to your small waistline. Or you could choose to draw the attention to your hips. Think about Jennifer Lopez, a famous pear who proudly put both of her best assets on display and single-handedly made curvy bodies and bigger butts a sexy statement during the time of the waif model being celebrated as the beauty standard. So, pear body shaped women, please know that your curves are drop-dead gorgeous, appreciate your shapely gifts!

Overall Strategy: Draw more attention to the upper body to bring you into balance with your lower body

Balancing Strategy: Add width to your shoulders; accentuate your waist to create a curvy balance

Color Strategy: Bright or light colors on top and dark colors on bottom will bring the eye up and add width to balance the top half of your body with your bottom half

Clothing Strategies:

Tops to Embrace

- Wearing bright colors on top draws attention upward

- Accessories around your face and shoulders will bring attention to your upper body

- Add shoulder width with V-shaped, strappy and strapless styles or detailed necklines

- Slim fitting tops define your waist and show off your small torso

- Wrap styles look beautiflly feminine, accentuate your upper body and waistline, and hide your small waist

Tops to Avoid

- Never wear anything boxy, it hides your waist and makes you look heavier

- Tops that end straight across the widest part of your hips add width

- Tops that end at or above your waist will make your hips look wider

Bottoms to Embrace

- Dark colored bottoms flatter wider hips

- Simple styles with very few details are slimming and create a sleek line

- Slim skirts ending below the knee or jagged hemlines flatter your shapely lower legs

- Pointy toe shoes with pants will make your legs look longer and slimmer

- Lean silhouettes are best; especially boot-cut pants

Bottoms to Avoid

- Details that add fullness—pleats, shirring, drawstrings, elastic, cargo pockets

- Tight pants and clingy bias cut skirts make the hips appear wider

- Pants with extreme shapes, tapering skinny or wide at the ankle widen hips to take your shape further out of balance

Pear Celebrities: Debra Messing, Jennifer Lopez, Kristen Davis, Kate Winslett, Michelle Obama, Cynthia Nixon, Kate Hudson, Oprah

HOURGLASS

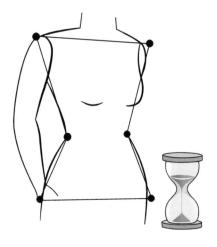

Your shoulders and hips are almost equal width. Your waist is clearly defined.

Zone of Beauty: Torso/Waistline

The iconic hourglass is the most desired body type for its proportional shape and strikingly feminine frame. In fact, only 8 percent of women have the hourglass shape! Just like the pear shape, your waistline is your best asset. In fact, you can consider framing your entire beautiful torso area as your spectacular Zone of Beauty. Because of your coveted balanced body, you have very few clothing limitations. Please feel free to proudly show off your naturally beautiful hourglass curves.

Overall Strategy: Accentuate your shape by emphasizing your waist

Balancing Strategy: Your bust and hips are the largest areas of your body—maximize your small torso

Color Strategy: Monochromatic colors add height and femininity to your shape

Clothing Strategies:

Tops to Embrace

- Wrap tops and dresses with torso emphasis flatter your small waist

- Any top or jacket with waist detail or cinched belts draw attention to your best asset

- V-necklines flatter and slim your décolletage, drawing attention to your bust

- Keep fabrics thin and lightweight to skim your curves and they'll flatter your feminine shape

Tops to Avoid

- Boxy styles hide your small waist and make you appear heavier

- Shirring below the bust adds bulk to your torso

- Bulky fabrics hide your shape and add weight

Bottoms to Embrace

- The best skirt style and shape is straight (pencil) and falls at the knee

- You can wear all pant shapes—skinny, boot and wide legs

Bottoms to Avoid

- You are blessed with the ideal shape and don't have any restrictions for bottoms

Hourglass Celebrities: Halle Berry, Kim Cattrall, Salma Hayek, Charlize Theron, Sandra Bullock, Eva Longoria, Shania Twain, Faith Hill, Sofia Vergara

APPLE

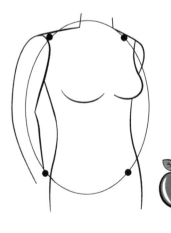

Your waist is not clearly defined. Your hips are narrow compared to the upper half of your body.

Zone of Beauty: Breasts or Legs

Of all the body types, I have found that apple-shaped women have the toughest time loving their bodies and feeling good about their shape. So, I'll spend more time with you

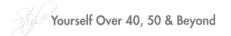

than the other body shapes to help you find the areas of your body you can embrace and feel good about. In our culture obsessed with slim bodies and curvy shapes, many apples feel left out and don't often see images in the media with their body type portrayed as beautiful. Yes, it's true that for apple shapes, you will have to work a bit harder to give yourself messages of self-appreciation and love that you are not getting from outside sources. However, I am here to share with you all the beautiful things that make your apple-shape body so special.

You are a womanly, voluptuous diva. Your fuller face gives you a youthful look. You are blessed with two beautiful Zones of Beauty. Your first Zone of Beauty, your full breasts, is the envy of all the other body shapes. While your fuller arms may be a source of self-consciousness, they are in perfect proportion with your upper body and are worthy of being shown and to be seen proudly in sleeveless styles. Your biggest challenge is your full midsection. When you are shopping, the stretchy, curvy styles that seem to be all around cause you much distress. Well, you can strategically camouflage your middle and choose to bring focus to your second Zone of Beauty, your slim, shapely legs.

One of my favorite examples of someone with an apple shape who chose her legs as her Zone of Beauty is Tina Turner. She cleverly and beautifully camouflaged her midsection with very short sparkly sheath dresses. She chose to proudly focus attention on an area of strength and beauty, her legs. Imagine the impact of her career if she had not confidently claimed her Zone of Beauty but instead chose to feel bad about her shape and did not strut her most positive stuff. It's time to accentuate the positives. Apples unite! Claim your beauty, choose your Zone, go out there and strut your stuff too!

Overall Strategy: Bring focus on top and show off your slim legs

Balancing Strategy: Minimize your midsection by drawing attention to your upper or lower body

Color Strategy: Dark colors on top help slim your full torso and small-scale dark prints give the illusion of a slimmer midsection

Clothing Strategies:

Tops to Embrace

- V-necklines lengthen the neck and slenderize your chest and shoulders

- Tunic styles and empire lines camouflage your larger middle

- Fabrics that skim your midsection will be much more flattering than anything tight

Tops to Avoid

- Clingy fabrics—avoid stretchy fabrics, especially with Lycra

- Bulky or chunky fabrics add weight

- Ruffles or fussy details around the neckline can overwhelm your frame

Bottoms to Embrace

- Skirts work well for you to show off your slim legs

- Pants that are full or fall straight balance your bigger middle

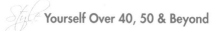

- Flat front pants, especially with a side zipper, flatten your middle

- Light bottoms make your lower body appear bigger to balance a larger midsection

Bottoms to Avoid

- Straight, tight-leg pants contrast your bigger middle and draw attention to it

- Pleats add bulk and make your middle appear larger

- Dark colors slim your bottom to take you body out of balance even more dramatically

Apple Celebrities: Chandra Wilson, Rosie O'Donnell, Angelina Jolie, Elizabeth Hurley, Tyra Banks, Tina Turner, Sigourney Weaver, Kathy Bates, Queen Latifah, Jennifer Hudson

RECTANGLE

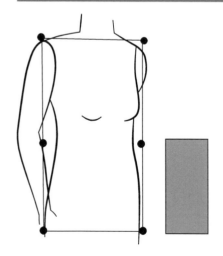

Your shoulders and hips are almost equal, and your waist is not clearly defined.

Zone of Beauty: Arms, Hips or Legs

You have a beautiful body shape with a parallel proportion that gives you a naturally athletic look. Your body frame is proportionally in line with all your body parts. Your biggest body challenge is creating curves to give you a more feminine shape. You have three Zones of Beauty to choose: your naturally toned arms, hips or legs. These choices will allow you to pick one to become your beautiful focal point and gives you a wide variety of fashion styles.

Overall Strategy: Create curves—add width to your upper and lower body to create the illusion of a smaller waist

Balancing Strategy: Keep the focus on the waist or upper body

Color Strategy: Prints and contrasting colors give the illusion of body shape

Clothing Strategies:

Tops to Embrace

- Strappy, strapless or form fitting tops look feminine on your narrow torso

- V-neck and low necklines widen your shoulders to make your waist look smaller

- Side shirring or dark side waist panels give the illusion of a smaller waist

- Layering, seaming, belted, shaped-waist styles create a shapely silhouette

- Bright accessories add bulk to give your narrow, straight frame more substance

Tops to Avoid

- Round or low scoop necklines are too bare if you have a small chest

- Vertical stripes and one color head to toe make you look too straight and narrow

- Short tops that end at your waist and loose, baggy tops do not add shape

Bottoms to Embrace

- You will look great in all jean styles, especially skinny jeans

- Pocket details add depth and give a curvy shape to your hips

- Wide belts define your waist

Bottoms to Avoid

- Boxy styles overwhelm your body—you need shaped garments

- Straight- or high-waist pants accentuate your straight shape

Rectangle Celebrities: Kelly Ripa , Carmen Diaz, Demi Moore, Sarah Jessica Parker, Gwen Stefani, Gweneth Paltrow, Nicole Kidman, Renee Zellwegger, Madonna, Cynthia Nixon, Dara Torres

INVERTED TRIANGLE

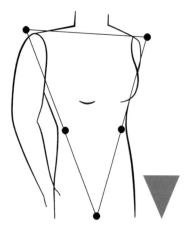

Your shoulders are wider than your hips.

Zone of Beauty: Hips

Your unique body shape—which starts broad at the top and narrows as you move down to your ankles—gives you a look of power and strength. To balance your shape, by placing emphasis on your narrow hips, you can get adventurous with designs, colors and styles on the bottom half of your body.

Overall Strategy: Move attention downward, towards your waist and hips

Balancing Strategy: Balance your upper body with your lower body by softening your shoulders—add width and volume to your lower body

Color Strategy: Dark colors on top, light colors on bottom

Clothing Strategies:

Tops to Embrace

• Wrap tops draw attention downward.

- Dark tops in simple designs minimize the width of your upper body

- Belted waist or tops with waist emphasis create the illusion of a smaller waist

- Soft and feminine layered tops give your waist definition

- Soft, smooth knits or woven fabrics with stretch glide over your body to add femininity and soften the wide lines of your shoulders

Tops to Avoid

- Shoulder-baring tops such as halters, strapless, boat neck or off the shoulder add width at the shoulders

- Boxy or full styles and exaggerated styling details—such as wide collars, lapels and epaulets—overwhelm your shape

- Tight, clingy or stiff fabrics without stretch and large-scale patterns add width

Bottoms to Embrace

- Light colors expand to make your lower body appear larger

- Details and shape such as wide-leg pants, full pleats, cargo pockets add width and fullness

Bottoms to Avoid

- Skinny jeans, pencil skirts or bottoms with a narrow shape exaggerate your narrow lower body and make your upper body appear larger

Inverted Triangle Celebrities: Gwyneth Paltrow, Renee Zellwegger, Naomi Campbell, Teri Hatcher, Demi Moore

Step 3:

UNDERSTANDING YOUR VERTICAL BODY

Once you have identified your horizontal body shape, the next important proportion to learn about is your vertical shape.

Two main descriptive shapes define the **Vertical Body Proportion**:

    1. Long Waist

    2. Short Waist

The ideal vertical body proportion is when your waist is perfectly centered between your head and feet. The placement of your waist affects how balanced your body looks. Choosing the right styles can bring your body into perfect symmetry.

Although the ideal waist placement is located at the center of your total body height, it is the placement of your waist on your torso that has the biggest impact on how your clothes fit and how you look in them. This measurement determines if your waist is short or long. There are several different ways to measure your vertical body measurements, but I prefer the simplest method.

To know if you have a short or long waist, you will need to find where your waist is placed on your torso in proportion to your shoulders and hips. If you were to merely measure the distance from your waist to your head—or from your waist to your feet— you would not have the most accurate reading of your vertical body proportions because these measurements do not reflect how your waist is placed on your torso. You might have long or short legs that affect the total measurement and the perception of your vertical body. So, our focus for now is simply on your torso.

If your waist is placed high or low on your torso, it will give your body the illusion of being out of balance in relation to the length of your legs. If your waist is placed high on your torso, you have a short waist. If your waist is placed low on your torso, you have a long waist. The general rule is:

Short waist = Long legs

Style Solution: Lengthen short torso to be in balance with long legs

Long waist = Short legs

Style Solution: Lengthen short legs to be in balance with long torso

Here's the bottom line: If your waist is located closer to your shoulders, you have a short waist. If your waist is located closer to your

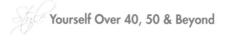

hips, you have a long waist. A body with a short waist gives the illusion of having a short torso and long legs. A body with a long waist gives the illusion of having a long torso and short legs.

How to measure the length of your waist:

Lay the tape measure at the center of your collarbone and extend it to the bottom of your crotch and write your total measurement in the spaces provided below.

Locate the smallest part of your waist on the tape measure and write the measurement of the length from the center of your collarbone to your waist.

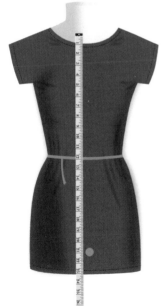

My total torso length is: _____

My waist length is: _____

Now, take the total measurement of your torso and divide it in half.

My half torso length is: _____

Is your Waist Length **Equal To** your Half Torso Length? If so, your vertical torso measurement is in perfect balance!

Is your Waist Length **Shorter Than** your Half Torso Length? If so, you have a short waist.

Is your Waist Length **Longer Than** your Half Torso Length? If so, you have a long waist.

My body has a _____ **waist**

Excellent! Now that you know your vertical body proportion, in the next step you'll get practical strategies to balance your body.

Step 4:

CLOTHING STRATEGIES TO BALANCE YOUR VERTICAL BODY

We've discussed the clothing strategies for your horizontal body in Step 2. Now, we'll address the clothing strategies for your vertical body to make sure you are in total balance.

CLOTHING STRATEGIES TO BALANCE YOUR BODY IF YOU HAVE A SHORT WAIST

The goal is to lengthen your shorter torso in proportion to your longer legs.

Tricks to Lengthen Your Torso:

- Add long, vertical lines to your torso. For example, wear tops that plunge vertically to give the illusion of torso length. This can be accomplished with deep V-neckline tops, long layered necklaces or long scarves.

- Tops that extend to your hipbone, long tops or tunics with a low-slung belt lengthen your torso

- Open, high, tall, dramatic collars or turtlenecks add length to your torso

- One long monochromatic block of color from top to bottom lengthens your torso

- Layered tops and vertical stripes add length to your torso

Avoid:

- Tucking tops into the waist of your pants, or wearing a top that ends at your waist, breaks your body in half and makes your legs appear shorter

- High, closed-in necklines shorten your torso

Tricks to Balance Your Lower Body:

- If you tuck your shirt into your pants or skirts, add a longer jacket or an open cardigan sweater to add length to your torso

- Wear longer untucked tops that fall to hipbone length to lengthen the look of your torso

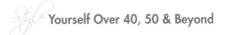

- Wear pants with a lower rise to add length to your torso

- A narrow belt, hip belt or a belt the same color as your pants will add length

CLOTHING STRATEGIES TO BALANCE YOUR BODY IF YOU HAVE A LONG WAIST

The goal is to shorten your long torso in proportion to your shorter legs.

Tricks to Shorten Your Torso:

- High, closed necklines shorten the torso

- Blouses and jackets with high belts work well to bring the waist up

- Empire tops bring the waist up

- Tuck tops into higher waist pants to shorten your midsection

- Wide waist belts shorten waist length

- Horizontal stripes add width and shorten length

Avoid:

- Drop waist tops or a tunic with a low slung belt—they will exaggerate your long torso

- Extending tops past your hipbone extends the length or your long torso

- Pants that are cropped or with cuffs—they shorten your legs

- Low rise pants—they lengthen your torso

Tricks to Balance Your Lower Body:

- Skirts are great choices because they add length, especially longer length skirts

- Choose pants with a higher rise, nice drape and long line

- Pant hems that extend to the floor to cover your shoes will lengthen your legs

- Heels lengthen your legs

- Wear shoes to match the color of your bottoms to lengthen your lower body

Part 3:

COMMUNICATE YOUR MESSAGE

Planning and preparing
to shop like a pro

Now that you have identified your Style Statement and how to flatter your shape, it's time to go shopping! But first, for you to have the best outcome, you'll need strategies to help you maximize your efforts. By taking the time to plan ahead, it will ensure you are focused towards making purchases that enhance and maximize your best assets.

Step 1: Decoding Fashion Terminology to Build a Balanced Wardrobe

Step 2: Release the Past and Embrace the New You!

Step 3: Find the Colors Aligned with Your Lifestyle

Step 4: Expand Your Clothing Choices with a Balanced Wardrobe

Step 5: Make a Big Impact with Foundation, Statement and Accent Pieces

Step 6: Taking Inventory of Your Layered Wardrobe

Step 7: Shopping with a Plan

Step 1:

DECODING FASHION TERMINOLOGY TO BUILD A BALANCED WARDROBE

I often hear references to fads and trends being used interchangeably. Part of the strategic shopping planning process requires a knowledge of the differences between fads and trends, and how they differ from classic styles. Understanding these differences will allow you to make the most informed buying decisions, and will help you to make and keep a closet that best represents your style.

Fads

A fad is introduced, quickly accepted, and fades fast. Fads are fun and can add a youthful energy to your style, but must be worn carefully to be age appropriate. A fad can be introduced as a new color, shape, style or detail. The life cycle of a fad is usually one to three years and develops very quickly in three phases.

The first phase of a fad begins with the introduction, where it is first seen and is highly sought after. You will see it on fashion runways, then in the media with celebrities wearing it and in magazines. It is initially offered at high prices with limited, exclusive accessibility. The second phase quickly penetrates the mainstream retail market, starting at high prices, then copied and sold at mid-level stores. Finally in the third phase, once it's available everywhere, it appears at discount stores for the lowest retail prices. This is when it loses its designer cachet, there is no longer a demand for it and the fad fades.

Fads in fashion often start from the streets. Designers and trend spotters are always looking for inspiration by observing people in everyday life engaged in activities that have a unique style expression. Fads are also inspired by styles from the past.

An example of a fashion fad that is recycled with a modern interpretation is fringe. It begins on the runways in designer collections. It is adopted and photographed by trendy fashionistas and quickly penetrates the mainstream market. It goes through the life cycle of a fad, all three phases, and then fades.

Trends

The life cycle of a trend starts as a mood, then shapes our attitudes, and is finally reflected as a style. A new trend is based on a societal mood that is the result of changes in our financial, social or political climates. Our mood shapes our attitude, and our attitude affects the way we choose to live. Our attitude also affects why, how and what we buy. Fashion is a reflection of these attitudes and designers create styles that cater to our new mindset.

The life span of a trend is not as definite as the life span of a fad. Trends could last from two–ten years. For instance, following the devastating events of 9/11, we felt shock and fear. Given this profound insecurity with a mood of uncertainty, we were seeking sources of comfort. Our attitude became all about feeling and staying safe, cocooning became the buzzword for comfort, and we were looking for ways to stay at home or close to the safety of home.

Uggs were introduced and were immediately embraced. The fluffy soft lining gave the secure feeling of home; they felt like wearing bedroom slippers or being wrapped in a cozy comforter. Even when venturing away from home, we could still have the safe, secure feeling of home with us. As the mood of uncertainty, doubt and fear decreased in intensity, so did our need for safety, security and cocooning, and the height of the trend for Uggs faded.

Classics

Classic styles are basic; they are enduring staples that never change. Classic styles flatter everyone, they have universal acceptance and are considered the basic foundation pieces of a wardrobe. A classic style has small design variations that reflect current trends, but the overall garment does not change.

For instance, a blazer is a classic wardrobe staple. The silhouette, fabric, color or collar changes to reflect current fashion trends, but the foundation of the item remains the same—an enduring classic.

Fashion Versus Style

Fashion is clothing; it entertains and entices, it is a reflection of our world at any current time. Fashion reflects the social, political and financial climate of the moment. Fashion is cyclical with offerings based on seasonal changes.

Style is personal and individualized. It is the unique expression of who you are on the inside and reflected on the outside to make a statement to the world.

Identity Versus Image

Your Identity is comprised of your values and personality . . . the essence of who you are.

Your Image is how others perceive you. Your style is a combination of your identity on the inside and your image on the outside.

Style Statement Dressing

Style Statement Dressing is an integration of your identity, image and how you live. When your Identity matches your Image and reflects how you live, you project a consistent authentic style that radiates confidence and creates a strong, compelling attraction.

FASHION DEFINITIONS TO REMEMBER

Fads are fun and short-lived; trends reflect attitudes; classics are enduring.

Designers create fashion; individuals create style.

Identity is internal; Image is external.

Step 2:

RELEASE THE PAST AND EMBRACE THE NEW YOU!

Another important step in the shopping planning process is to start with an organized closet. By organizing, reducing and releasing clutter, you can gain a feeling of lightness and clarity. As we go through changes during this transitional phase of life over 40, cleaning your closet can serve as a surprisingly powerful emotional experience that allows you to release and embrace.

Releasing can help make peace with things you may be holding on to from the past that could be holding you back. Going though all the clothes in your closet may reveal many items that you haven't worn in years—or items that you wear just because you have worn them for so many years. If this is true for you, it means that there is something you are holding on to for emotional reasons. It could be that certain garments remind you of good times in the past, or times you looked great, or maybe even a gift from someone special. But, if those garments are old, and especially if you haven't worn them in a while, let them go! Release the garment and the emotion! You may feel the need to grieve the loss of these garments, perhaps even cry, but do so with the knowledge that you are creating a clearing for something new and wonderful.

Once you have released, you can embrace who you are today and who you want to be tomorrow. You will discover a new capacity to visualize yourself in a future containing possibilities that you may have only got a glimpse of in the past. Embracing means an ability to own dreams and goals grounded in the reality of who you are. If you are able to accept yourself and make these emotional adjustments, you will find that you will feel happier and more content than at any other time in your life.

What I am trying to convey is how much the seemingly mundane task of closet cleansing may prove to be a cathartic experience that could bring a sense of comfort and security. Spending time in our closet is something we do every day, and it can kick-start the day by either triggering an emotionally negative feeling or a wonderfully positive feeling of well-being that comes from loving self-care. An organized closet may be just the thing you need to start each day feeling good.

When you have successfully cleaned your closet and released, you will be able to embrace:

- Eliminating garments that do not accurately or appropriately express you

- A feeling of accomplishment and control in your life—the current state of your closet is a reflection of your state of mind in other areas

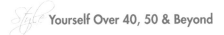

- Strategically shaping your image by handpicking items that will be worn to proudly communicate who you are to the world

- Quickly finding what you need to make getting dressed simpler and stress free

CLEANING YOUR CLOSET

To clean your closet, you'll need:

A Good Mood: Find time on your schedule when you can anticipate feeling good; a good attitude about your body and a time when you will have high energy.

Uninterrupted Time: When you have <u>at least</u> four hours without time pressure.

Privacy: Structure your time to remove distractions or interruptions; this is precious time for you to invest in yourself.

Tools: You'll need good lighting, hangers, a full-length mirror and a step stool (optional, but handy if you have high shelves to reach). Also optional, but handy, is a collapsible rolling rack to use when you move garments out of your closet for review; otherwise you can just place the garments on your bed. You may also need storage bins for anything you need to remove from your closet that is not essential for getting dressed every day, but need to be stored elsewhere.

Food: Eat a light meal before starting, have a snack and plenty of water on hand.

Honesty: This is a time for you to have tough love with yourself and take the long view of your future. Many people have a difficult time with change and releasing—they have emotional attachments with many clothing items—or some may feel purging is being wasteful. Sometimes an emotion may come up when getting rid of a garment that does not fit; it may feel like you are giving up hope of losing weight. If you are having an especially difficult time parting with your weight-loss goal clothes, here's a suggestion that may work for you. Take the goal clothes and put them in a special box and write a loving note to yourself about how you will feel when you reach your goal and fit into the clothes. When you reach your weight goal, you can open the box of new clothes and celebrate your success.

If you have challenges in any of these areas, it may be helpful to make a pact with yourself to be reassured that these are positive changes. Remember that it is necessary to release so that you can make room for all the wonderful things that lie ahead. If you anticipate you will be having difficulty making decisions to release, invite a trusted, honest friend or family member who has a realistic perspective to nudge you along.

Music: Choose music that makes you feel good; it will keep your energy high and spirits up.

Bags: You will be filling four bags—one for the dry cleaners, one for charity or to give away to friends, one for the trash and one to take to a tailor for alterations. If you do not have a reliable tailor, start by asking three stylish friends for a referral or go to your local dry cleaners.

Hangers: Even your hangers need to be organized! It is important to have the proper hangers in your closet—not only to create the

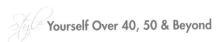

order you need, but for your clothes to maintain their proper shape. They will make your closet look like a beautifully organized fashion boutique. You can choose matching molded plastic tubular hangers or slim-line styles, especially if space is at a premium.

You will need five types of hangers:

1. Basic hangers for tops and blouses

2. Hangers with grips or grooves to hold tops with thin straps in place

3. Pant hangers with clips

4. Heavy-duty hangers for suit jackets and coats

5. Belt and scarf racks or hooks

Supply Resources: Some of my favorite retailers for closet supplies are Target, The Container Store, Hold Everything, Ikea, Target, Home Depot, and Bed, Bath & Beyond.

My Commitment to Cleaning My Closet

I will clean my closet on this date _____

To be completely prepared for my closet cleaning, I will have the supplies listed below no later than _____

My Supply List

Hangers	**Supplies**
__Basic with grooves for straps	__Full-length Mirror
__Basic for tops	__Step Stool (optional)
__Pant hangers	__Rolling Rack (optional)
__Heavy-duty for jackets	__Trash Bags
__Belt rack	__Snacks
__Scarf rack	__Music

Decision Making Criteria

Begin your closet cleaning process in one of two ways: by emptying your entire closet or by removing clothing in categories (all tops, pants, etc.). Begin making decisions one category at a time. If you need help with decision making, here are a few clothing guidelines to help make the process successful.

As you review each garment, decide in which one of the four stacks it belongs:

1. To keep

2. To give away

3. To have altered

4. To throw away

Be decisive; do not create a maybe stack.

Now, it's time to get started. Review and critique each garment. Be prepared to try on some of the clothes to make sure it meets the following criteria:

Style Statement Criteria

Does it communicate my authentic Style Statement?

Yes   No

Is the garment in current style; is it modern or an enduring classic?

Yes   No

Have I worn this item within the last five years? (If not, let it go!)

Yes   No

Is this a seasonal or sentimental item? (If yes, it should not be in your closet—place it elsewhere for storage.)

Yes   No

Body Shape Criteria

Does it balance and flatter my horizontal body shape?

Yes   No

Does is balance and flatter my vertical body frame?

Yes   No

Fit Criteria

Does this garment fit and flatter me right now? (Release the habit of buying or keeping garments as an incentive, or to fit when you lose weight.)

Yes   No

Tops

Does the top lie smoothly or properly against my neckline?

Yes   No

Do the shoulders/armholes have proper placement across my shoulders?

Yes   No

Does the top lie smoothly across my bust, with no pulls or gaps between buttons?

Yes   No

Does the top gently curve around my bust at the underarm, without extra fabric, tightness or pulling?

Yes   No

Does the short-sleeve hemline end at an age-appropriate, flattering length?

Yes   No

Bottoms

Do the pants zip and button comfortably?

Yes   No

Is the front rise excessively high or low?

Yes   No

Does the front rise fit properly, and not too low or tight in the crotch?

Yes   No

Does the back rise fit properly when standing, gently molding around the curve of my backside without pulling tightly across or digging in?

Yes   No

Does the back rise fit properly when sitting, appropriately covering my backside or is it too shallow revealing too much?

Yes   No

Do the pant legs fall gently to the floor without pulling tightly at the thighs, knees or twisting around the legs?

Yes   No

Do the pant legs cover the back of the bottom of my shoe?

Yes   No

Fabric Criteria

Are there any snags, pulls, tears or holes, or pilling (fuzz balls)?

Yes   No

Has the garment stretched and lost recovery?

Yes   No

Does the garment have any permanent stains or has it faded?

Yes   No

Is the fabric high quality and communicate the right age-appropriate image?

Yes   No

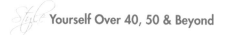

Accessories, Undergarments and Sleepwear

Go through the same process with your accessories, undergarments and sleepwear as you do with your other clothing items. Go through your drawers and take out your undergarments and sleepwear. Take out your shoes, purses, scarves, belts, hats and jewelry to give them the same singular scrutiny as your clothing, and follow the criteria list as it applies.

GETTING YOUR NEW CLOSET IN ORDER

It's time to start rebuilding your closet now that you have finished clearing the clothes from it. But first, make sure it has been completely cleared—that means all clothes, shoes, hats, boxes, bags and anything else you have previously stored in there.

Think about your new closet as a beautiful fashion boutique. You can set the stage for it to give you a good feeling every day you go into it—the same good feeling you get when you walk into a beautiful store to browse. Imagine your new closet as a place for renewal. Every time you step into it, you are reminded of the great work you did to get it there. You can see everything in it, and all of the items fit you and your style perfectly. Getting dressed is now stress-free and fast!

Some of the elements that add ambience to the closet of your dreams are:

- Nice lighting

- Matching hangers

- Shelves for folded items

- An unobstructed and clean floor

- Pretty baskets for any loose items

- Proper storage for accessories, shoe boxes or racks

Once everything has been completely cleared, take inventory to make sure you have all the items you need for the closet you really want. Before you begin to put clothes back into your closet, give it a thorough cleaning by vacuuming and dusting. There may be something else you need since you first started—you may need brighter lighting, or you may want to add a shelf. Take notes and replenish your supplies later.

Now you can put everything back into your clean closet, one category at a time. Organize it carefully, hang garments in the same direction and group like colors together from light to dark. Carefully place folded garments on the shelves. Place accessories and shoes together and easily in sight. Once you have put everything away, you can see what you have left and what you need to buy.

The balance of this section will take you through several steps that will create a balanced wardrobe to accommodate the reality of your current style and life.

Step 3:

FIND THE COLORS ALIGNED
WITH YOUR STYLE STATEMENT

Color is a powerful means of expression. All colors have meanings that provoke emotion and communicate an unspoken statement about who you are. It gives us a peek into your personality.

The meaning of color is so powerful that it can produce unconscious physical and emotional reactions. It can excite, calm, draw you towards or move you away from it.

Imagine how you could do the same and use color to positively influence those around you, too. You can intentionally choose a color to provoke an emotional response and set the tone for an interaction. Now, that's the power of color!

The best use of color is to align it to your personality to create the most consistent and comprehensive message. By understanding the underlying meaning of colors and how they can affect others, you can make style choices with thoughtful intention. The outcome is a powerful and accurately personal expression of your essence from the inside out.

Color Questionnaire

The following questionnaire will help you identify your Signature Colors. Review the list and circle the attributes that most accurately describe you; then total your score for each.

Color 1

Trustworthy	Dependable	Committed	Loyal
Conservative	Responsible		Total: _____

Color 2

Relaxed	Playful	Tranquil	Youthful
Thoughtful	Expressive		Total: _____

Color 3

Powerful	Responsible	Competent	Calm
Conscientious	Intuitive		Total: _____

Color 4

Healthy	Relaxing	Hopeful	Tolerant
Harmonious	Generous		Total: _____

Color 5

Optimistic	Vibrant	Enlightened	Fun
Inspiring	Communicative		Total: _____

Color 6

Mysterious	Strong-Willed	Powerful	Creative
Disciplined	Independent		Total: _____

Color 7

Warm	Spontaneous	Decisive	Active
Experimental	Positive		Total: _____

Color 8

Exciting	Energetic	Protective	Stimulating__
Confident	Enthusiastic		Total: _____

Color 9

Feminine	Romantic	Sensitive	Loving
Emotional	Nurturing		Total: _____

Color 10

Spiritual	Perceptive	Reassuring	Respectful
Sophisticated	Strong		Total: _____

Color 11

Stable	Reliable	Patient	Warm
Approachable	Practical		Total: _____

Color 12

Open-minded   Devoted   Faithful   Peaceful

Honest   Focused   Total: _____

Color Totals

Color 1: ___   Color 2: ___   Color 3: ___   Color 4: ___

Color 5: ___   Color 6: ___   Color 7: ___   Color 8: ___

Color 9: ___   Color 10: ___   Color 11: ___   Color 12: ___

Once you have marked your answers, find the colors with the top three highest totals. Now list those color numbers in order of highest to lowest. These top three colors most accurately express your personality—these are your Primary Colors.

Color Number: ____   Color Number: ____   Color Number: ____

Now list your next three highest ranking colors. These are your Secondary Colors. They also express your personality, and you'll use them to coordinate with your primary color palette.

Color Number: ____   Color Number: ____   Color Number: ____

Your Signature Colors

So, which colors did you choose? The combination of your primary colors and your secondary colors combine to form your Signature Color Palette. Review the following chart to reveal your color choices, their attributes and effect. After you've identified your primary colors, we'll discuss how you can use them, as well as other colors, to best express yourself to make the most powerful Style Statement.

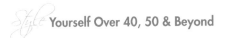

Color	Attributes	Physical Effect
1 Navy	Trustworthy Dependable Committed Conservative Loyal Responsible	❖ Communicates more peacefully ❖ Develops deeper faith and trust ❖ Overcomes loneliness, depression or shyness ❖ Suggests expertise and competence
2 Turquoise	Relaxed Playful Tranquil Youthful Thoughtful Expressive	❖ Enhances communication ❖ Inspires independent creative thoughts and feelings ❖ Facilitates telepathic communication ❖ Allows better self-expression
3 Blue	Powerful Responsible Competent Conscientious Intuitive Calm	❖ Encourages more powerful communication ❖ Inspires confidence and trust ❖ Ignites spiritual awakening ❖ Restores a sense of calm
4 Green	Healthy Relaxing Hopeful Harmonious Tolerant Generous	❖ Offers a sense of renewal, self-control and harmony ❖ Helps alleviate depression, nervousness and anxiety ❖ Forges friendship and tolerance ❖ Creates a sense of harmony
5 Yellow	Optimistic Vibrant Enlightened Inspiring Communicative Fun	❖ Stimulates mental processes and nervous system ❖ Activates memory ❖ Accelerates the thinking process ❖ Enhances clarity, focus and decision making

Color	Attributes	Physical Effect
6 Black	Mysterious Strong-Willed Powerful Disciplined Independent Creative	❖ Evokes a sense of potential and possibility ❖ Encourages order and self-control ❖ Suggests style and creativity ❖ Inspires a feeling of elegance
7 Orange	Warm Spontaneous Decisive Experimental Positive Active	❖ Stimulates activity ❖ Radiates warmth and energy ❖ Attracts attention ❖ Encourages socialization
8 Red	Exciting Energetic Enthusiastic Protective Stimulating Confident	❖ Stimulates energy; can increase blood pressure and pulse ❖ Encourages action, confidence and visibility ❖ Boosts physical vitality, sexual drive ❖ Sparks a spirit of adventure and certainty
9 Pink	Feminine Romantic Sensitive Emotional Nurturing Loving	❖ Encourages kindness and generosity ❖ Cultivates relationships ❖ Develops powers of intuition and creativity ❖ Promotes self-acceptance

Color	Attributes	Physical Effect
10 Purple	Spiritual Perceptive Reassuring Sophisticated Respectful Strong	❖ Offers a sense of spirituality ❖ Calms the mind and nerves ❖ Encourages creativity ❖ Aids in recovery from illness
11 Brown	Stable Reliable Patient Approachable Practical Warm	❖ Creates a sense of orderliness ❖ Fosters a connection to the earth ❖ Inspires structure and stability ❖ Represents a feeling of dependability and trustworthiness
12 White	Open-minded Devoted Faithful Peaceful Honest Focused	❖ Aids mental clarity ❖ Enables fresh beginnings ❖ Promotes physical health and healing ❖ Suggests future/technology

Your top three colors are your **Primary Color Palette.** Record your responses below. Then do the same for your next three highest ranking colors—this is your **Secondary/Accent Color Palette.**

Primary Color Palette	Secondary Color Palette

As you think about these six colors: Are any of these colors currently in your closet? Do you naturally gravitate towards wearing any of these colors?

If you are not currently wearing any of these colors or do not own them, this may be a great time for you to consider how you could incorporate them into your wardrobe.

You could choose one of your top three primary colors as the base of your outfit, and one of the colors from your secondary color palette to coordinate as an accent.

Whatever decision you make about how to wear one of your **Signature Colors,** the best thing to do is integrate it into your wardrobe, and start making conscious choices to show your personality.

Additionally, you could choose one color to "own" as your signature for business occasions and a different one for your personal time. There are a few questions to ask yourself when making the decision about the best color choice for personal, business and love life.

- Does it stand out in the way I want to make an impression?

- Are there various shades within this color that could make the most impact and be memorable?

- How appropriate is it for the occasion?

- How does this color make me feel?

- Will it be a priority for me to be more comfortable or to put others at ease?

Communicating with Color

You've now identified your Signature Colors; however, I'm not suggesting you should be confined to only those. This is simply a way to give you consistency in your wardrobe. It will help you create a foundation that expresses your personality most accurately and vividly.

Now that you know your Signature Colors, you can be mindful of using them to guide you when shopping. By wearing your signature colors, this can help you further communicate your unique style.

Below is a list of each color with their unique attributes and suggestions about how to further incorporate them into your wardrobe. You can make your color choice based on the intention and outcome you want for different occasions.

Red: Associated with passion, excitement and confidence, wearing red can increase your energy and get the hearts of others pounding. Depending on your circumstance, wear all-over red with caution.

In most circumstances, red is best worn as an accent to give your outfit an exciting punch of color. If you're drawn to red but feeling a bit shy about wearing it from head to toe, try deeper shades such as wine or burgundy. These shades can still bring all the drama with less intensity.

Orange: This is a color that attracts attention, which is the reason orange vests are worn by road workers (so we'll see them) and the same reason employees at Home Depot wear them. We can quickly and easily spot them down the store aisles.

If you want to be the center of attention, orange would be your choice. It is best worn as a color accent or within a print surrounded by other colors.

Pink: Associated with femininity and romance, pink is the choice when you want to show your softer side. Most men would cringe at the idea of wearing pink, so this is an ultra-feminine statement, and it signals that you are nurturing and sensitive.

Stronger shades of pink are stunning when worn as a sold-color dress. Softer shades of pink are relaxing and approachable—a perfect choice when you want someone to feel at ease. Pink is beautiful as a top or scarf around your face. It is also the best shade of lipstick for all skin tones—it gives a soft and pretty look.

Purple: The color of sophistication and royalty, purple has an elegance unrivaled by any other color. It is a relatively rare color in nature, which makes it especially striking and memorable. It is stunning in all shades, from soft pastels to jewel tones. It is also beautifully worn in all fabric textures—from a matte wool suit to a shiny silk blouse. Enjoy being a head-turner in all shades of purple.

Blue: Blue is the number one color and is universally loved by all. It is easy to wear and flatters everyone. It has a calming effect and is best worn when you want to facilitate communication, be more approachable and thought of as sincere.

However, dark shades of blue, such as navy, are more powerful than the lighter shades and will give you an air of depth, expertise and stability. It also suggests loyalty and protection—the reason it is worn by law enforcement. It would be a great choice for an interview.

Yellow: This is the color of happiness and optimism—the way we feel when the sun is shining brightly. If you want to light up a room and bring in the sunshine, wear yellow and you will attract attention and create a vibrant, happy aura. It also can accelerate

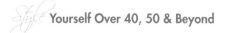

the thinking process and activate memory—these attributes are the reason pencils, Post-its and legal pads are yellow.

Yellow is the most challenging color for the eye to process. It can be overwhelming and best worn in smaller scale clothing items. Yellow does not easily work with all skin tones, so make sure it is a complementary color against your face. Otherwise, keep it to the accessories. If yellow is a flattering color for you, enjoy wearing it to social events and enjoy spreading happiness!

Green: This is the color of harmony, health and well-being. If you want to project a sense of balance with an earthy wholesomeness, then this would be your best choice. Green is easy on the eye and is the most common color seen in the beauty of nature. It can easily translate to enhance beauty when worn next to the skin. Find your best shade of green and wear it against your face to facilitate friendship and harmonious interactions.

Green is also a symbol of wealth and prosperity, which is the reason it is the color of money. If you want to project success, a deeper shade of green would be an excellent choice for a business meeting.

Black: An elegant color, black evokes independence and creativity. Wearing all black can be mysterious and dramatic. If you want to soften your look, you can pair black with soft pastels for a more feminine feeling. White paired with black evokes formality and is striking with its high contrast. Bright colors with black are more creative and playful.

Brown: This is the color of nature, grounded and deep. By wearing brown, you show that you are a person who is approachable, trustworthy and dependable.

You can experiment with different shades of brown. Khaki gives a classic look. Camel is sophisticated and brings even more depth when worn head to toe or paired with dark brown or black. Dark browns are the most stable and have an earthy reliability. They look best from head to toe during cooler temperatures. The warmth of brown worn against the face is flattering and facilitates a feeling of trust—perfectly appropriate for business settings or beginning new relationships.

White: Wearing all white can suggest a pulled-together perfection. It can have an open-minded fresh appeal with an aura of purity and honesty. In contrast, all white can also appear unfriendly, cold and clinical—the reason it is the choice for hospitals. So based on the fabric and setting, use your best judgment when wearing all white.

White worn as a secondary color is a perfect contrast to every color. It is a beautiful color for every complexion, adding light to the face, which can soften fine lines and give you the appearance of looking years younger.

Making Conscious and Strategic Color Choices

There are many times when we make unconscious color choices with clothing decisions and purchases. Our mood has much to do with the colors we choose and ultimately decide to buy. Many experts believe we feel colors before we see them. Ideally, for the most powerful and total expression of your Signature Style, you will become attuned to your signature colors, their attributes and how they communicate, which will allow you to make thoughtful, conscious choices.

Corporations understand the power of color and use it to their advantage. Color has a language all its own. It is used as to make products more appealing or to attract attention and, hopefully, lead to a purchase. Color power is so profound that experts in all industries use the psychology of color and "sensory branding" (the study of how appealing they can make their product to you). By using color, they can fine tune it to make it look good and feel good. Also, retail interior designers use color to cause us to linger or leave an environment.

For instance, in some restaurants, color is used to create a calm and relaxing environment so you will stay and, in turn, increase the amount you will spend. In many fast food restaurants, color is used to appear friendly and inviting, but not enough for you to linger—you subconsciously feel the desire to leave. It is to their benefit to serve as many customers as possible, so a high table turnover is encouraged.

Many companies use color as a branding strategy. It is used as a way to differentiate themselves from competitors and to communicate their brand personality, values and attributes. Color can increase brand recognition up to 80 percent! It has been stated that some purchase decisions were made within 90 seconds and based on color alone. Here are examples of companies "owning" a color as a defining brand strategy and communicating their personality:

UPS
Color: Brown
Meaning: Dependable, trustworthy, protective

Target
Color: Red
Meaning: Fun, exciting, unexpected

Home Depot
Color: Orange
Meaning: New, experimental, active

In the way large corporations have used color as a language to communicate their personality and make a memorable brand statement, you can do the same. Now that you have the knowledge of your primary and secondary colors and attributes, you can begin to think about how you would wear them to affect your mood, integrate into your personal style or affect the outcome of your environment.

As an example, when it was time to make color choices for the outfit on my book cover, I began by getting clear about my intention and the intended outcome. My intention was to show my expertise, corporate experience and fashion style. I also wanted to show my personality—a casual person who is friendly, open and approachable.

I prioritized my list based on the attributes I wanted to lead with. I thought about how quickly someone glances at a book cover and makes an instantaneous decision to explore further. I decided my priority was to lead with my professional attributes. I wanted someone to know they were in the capable hands of an expert. In addition, I wanted them to know I was a casual person, someone who they would feel comfortable with discussing the issues of style; so a casual, friendly approach was very important to me and is completely authentic to who I am. The outcome I wanted was for women to pick up the book, find it helpful and buy it.

For my color choices, I chose black as the primary color. It evokes a feeling of potential and possibility. These are the leading outcomes I wanted women to feel and, personally, wanted to project.

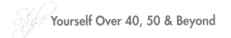

For a secondary color under the jacket, I wanted to lighten and brighten the black. I chose white, as opposed to pink, which didn't bring enough contrast when paired with black. White would brighten my face and had the attributes of being open minded and enables fresh beginnings. These attributes are a perfect match for a woman over 40 who wants to re-ignite her style!

With this in mind, you can use color to shape or change perception. Think about different circumstances or scenarios and how you could use color to create the most desirable outcome.

If you were going on a date, what is your intention and what is the outcome you want? If you choose red, it could produce a reaction and perception different than if you chose to wear a beautiful shade of blue.

At a networking event, you might think about the colors that represent your brand or the colors that facilitate interaction, or the colors that will make you appear more approachable.

There are many times when getting dressed, we gravitate to colors that reflect our mood. Sometimes this is a conscious decision and many times it is unconscious. We may be affected hormonally by color choices or how we feel about the size of our body. For whatever reason you have decided to use color, consciously or not, it is best used when you bring the meaning of color to your consciousness so that when you are making clothing decisions, you are doing so with a sense of purpose and intention.

Color can be used strategically to attract or detract attention to our bodies. It can be used to highlight and enhance your Zone of Beauty. You can use dark colors to deemphasize areas of your body. You can also use a dark color as a way to add contrast or draw more attention to an area of your body.

You can thoughtfully use color to bring your style into clearer focus. So the next time you get dressed, I encourage you to take a strategic approach by using color. It starts by getting clear on defining your intention followed by understanding your intended outcome. Once you have defined this, then you can choose on the most conscious and knowledgeable level to enhance your Signature Style.

Step 4:

EXPAND YOUR CLOTHING CHOICES WITH A BALANCED WARDROBE

Identifying the way you spend your time each day will help establish purchase priorities to create a Balanced Wardrobe that meets the needs of your Style Statement. The proportion of clothing you buy and own should be in direct relationship to how you live. For instance, if you work from home, are a stay-at-home mom or retired, your priorities would be very different from a woman who is working outside the home.

The goal is to create a balanced wardrobe based on how you spend the majority of your time. A common problem of a wardrobe that is out of balance is a career woman who has built a work wardrobe filled with beautiful suits but has an underdeveloped selection of weekend leisure clothes. When she is ready to enjoy an activity outside of work, she can become frustrated while getting dressed due to the lack of comparable casual choices. She is used to looking polished when she gets dressed for work but does not feel the same pride when getting dressed for leisure or weekend activities.

The following questionnaire will help you get a snapshot of how you spend your time. It will help you prioritize your purchases to maintain a proportionally balanced wardrobe that matches your Style Statement.

LIFESTYLE ASSESSMENT

Circle only one choice in each category below that most closely represents how you live:

Work Life

    A. I do not work

    B. I work from home

    C. I work outside the home

Home Life

    A. I am a mother with young children

    B. I am a mother with teen or older children

    C. I do not have children at home or I am not a mother

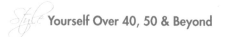

Social Life

  A. I do very little socializing

  B. I actively socialize with a close circle of family and friends

  C. Most of my socializing is career focused networking

Leisure Life

  A. I enjoy quiet home-based hobbies

  B. I spend most of my leisure time with outdoor recreational and sporting events

  C. I enjoy spending time with friends at a variety of social activities

In the space below, mark how many times you circled A, B or C.

Your Totals: A._____ B._____ C._____

Most of my answers are _____

If most of your answers are:

A. Home Based

You enjoy a quiet life close to home wearing casual, comfortable clothing that makes you feel relaxed. **Foundation Clothing** should be your first priority for building a strong and practical wardrobe. This will give you all the choices you need to look and feel your best.

You can begin to build your wardrobe by following the **Foundation List** in the next section. It will be important to start right at the top of the list and buy a good bra. This will form the essential base you will need to create a flattering look for all your casual tops. Adding more comfortable leisure pants to your list will give you enough choices to be comfortable around the house, and look pulled together when you go out.

B. On the Move

You are active and enjoy spending time with friends at home and activities away from home. You need a wardrobe that is flexible and meets your needs for comfort, yet with enough fashion for socializing.

Once you have an adequate **Foundation** wardrobe established, making the **Statement** category a priority is a great place for you to focus. This category will meet your Lifestyle needs to ensure you have enough variety of fashion choices to take you from inside the home to outside activities.

C. Socializer

Your life is highly social and active. A polished presence is essential for your Style Statement. Once your **Foundation** and **Statement** categories are adequately established, a focus towards building a

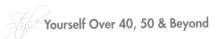

large variety in the **Accent** category will help you achieve your style goals.

Unique and powerful accent pieces will give your outfits a highly individualized appearance and create a signature style. However, building a strong **Accent** category takes time—the power pieces that work with your Style Statement take time and patience to find just the right choices.

Step 5:

MAKE A BIG IMPACT WITH FOUNDATION, STATEMENT AND ACCENT PIECES

Foundation Pieces are basic garments that are worn alone or form the "foundation" to layer pieces from other apparel categories. They are the most enduring and essential part of your wardrobe.

Statement Pieces are unique garments that authentically project your style through design details and express your unique style statement. This is where color, texture, fabric and garment details come together to represent you and express the essence of your Style Statement.

Accent Pieces are accessories that punctuate your outfit and style—they express, define or give your outfit a finished look. They are the details that define you, catch attention, serve as conversation starters or complete your outfit. They can also camouflage or accentuate your features, and can strategically direct attention to the area where you want someone to look.

Putting It All Together

By incorporating all three aspects of your style profile into your clothing choices to include your Style Statement, Body Shape and Lifestyle, you will more easily and fully express yourself with confidence and authenticity. The additional benefits of following this strategy are:

- You will project a consistent image to gain trust and attraction by dressing in your unique Style Statement.

- Your body appears taller, slimmer and in perfect balance by dressing for your unique Body Shape.

- You'll reduce stress by easily finding clothes in your closet.

For you to begin putting it all together, combine your complete style profile to include your Style Statement, Body Shape and Lifestyle:

My Style Statement: _____

My Horizontal Body Shape: _____

My Vertical Body Shape: _____

My Lifestyle: _____

The example below represents how you can select and combine pieces to complete an outfit in your style profile.

Style Statement: <u>Chic</u>

Body Shape: <u>Hourglass/Short Waist</u>

Daily Life: <u>Out and About</u>

Foundation

Undergarment: A strategically chosen foundation outfit starts with a bra that has been professionally fitted to give you the proper support and slimming line.

Top: A black, V-neck T-shirt that extends slightly past the hipbone to give the torso the added length it needs to extend the short waist.

Statement

Pants: Fabulous fitting dark-wash jeans that have a lower rise to lengthen the shorter torso. The jeans taper beautifully to the hemline, covering the shoes and flattering your longer legs.

Jacket: A blazer in a unique color with an interesting design detail transforms the T-shirt from a simple foundation piece to a unique statement that conveys your style.

Accent

Accessories: Jewelry becomes the strong accent with a bold, chunky necklace in a unique color as the focal point that draws attention to the face and transforms a basic foundation outfit into a personal style expression.

Your closet will be in complete balance when each of the three areas—Foundation, Statement and Accent pieces— are prioritized in direct proportion to your Lifestyle.

Step 6:

TAKING INVENTORY OF
YOUR LAYERED WARDROBE

**Now that you have cleared your closet and assessed your
Style Statement needs, it is time to take inventory of
what you have and where you need to replenish.** Review
the three category checklists below and mark the items you have in
your closet. Then go back and review the list to see the items you
will need to buy. These will be the areas where you may need to fill
in and buy new items. It is best to start with the category that was
identified in the Lifestyle Assessment as your area of focus and priority. You'll find a complete list in Part 5 for you to copy and place
in your closet.

THE FOUNDATION WARDROBE

Undergarments

Bras are one of the essential items that don't get enough attention for the degree of importance and impact they have on your style. You could be wearing the most beautiful top but if you are wearing a poor fitting bra that causes your breasts to sag or if your bra strap is too tight and creating back fat, your style is abruptly halted. My general shopping rule is that most women over 40 benefit from a well-made push-up bra to give added support (unless you have had augmentation). Hormonal fluctuations can cause changes in the shape and size of your breasts—this is the reason bras will need to be regularly updated for proper fit.

It is important to get professionally fitted to make sure you are buying the right bra size. You can walk into any bra department and ask to be fitted free of charge. However, if you would prefer the convenience and privacy of fitting yourself at home, you will find complete instructions for the most accurate and professional results on my website. Please visit www.TheStyleConcierge.com/findyourbrasize.

Shapers can perform miracles under your clothes—they can either be used to reshape your body or give a smooth appearance for your clothes to drape beautifully. There are many types of shapers with different levels of tension to hold you in and they are available at many price points. You can choose to buy a lightweight camisole shaper to control your midsection and wear it under your slimmer fitting garments on most days, or use shapers with more control for special occasions.

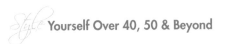

Shaper panties are essential under lightweight, knit, tight or light colored pants. They eliminate panty lines, conceal cellulite and give your body a smooth and sleek appearance.

Bras

Seamless Push-Up
__2 Black __2 Nude

Strapless
__1 Nude

Racer Back
__1 Nude

Shapers

Midsection/Torso
__1 Nude

Hips and Thighs
__1 Nude

Tops

Foundation tops are the indispensable items in your closet that get the most wear. They are worn alone or layered, and help extend the range of your fashion options. When selecting foundation tops, it is important to be mindful of the body shape guidelines to make sure you keep your body in balance. When you find a brand that fits you perfectly, it's a good idea to buy it in several colors.

Camisoles
__1 Black __1 White __Colors

Tank Tops
__1 Black __1 White __Colors

Short Sleeve T-Shirts
__1 Black __1 White

Long Sleeve T-Shirts
__1 Black __1 White

Pants

Foundation pants also get frequent wear compared to any other clothing category. This is where you can take your time to find the perfect fit; you will get so much wear out of them that you will feel like they are your uniform pants.

Foundation jeans should be a mid-tone to dark wash. The style should be basic and the fit should follow body shape guidelines.

Slacks also follow the body shape guidelines; for instance, pear-shaped bodies avoid light colored pants, but inverted triangles and rectangles can embrace them.

Your lounge pants are primarily worn around the house or for running errands in the neighborhood. They are most comfortable when they are slightly loose, and feel soft and cozy against your skin. The fabric is a very personal preference—some women prefer knit, jersey or fleece fabrics, while others prefer comfortable denim.

Lounge Pants
__1 Black __Colors

THE STATEMENT WARDROBE

Tops

Statement tops move beyond basic neckline designs and fabrics. They are unique through design details in fabric, embellishment, neckline shape or silhouette.

Short Sleeve T-Shirts
__3 Solid Colors
__1 Patterns/Prints

Long Sleeve T-Shirts
__3 Solid Colors
__1 Patterns/Prints

Shirts/Blouses
__3 Solid Colors __2 Patterns/Prints

Bottoms

Statement pants get the most frequent wear compared to any other clothing category. This is where you should take your time to find the perfect fit. When selecting your statement jeans, follow your body shape guidelines first, then the styling according to your Style Statement. Pants also follow the same body shape guidelines. For instance, a great looking pair of cropped khaki cargo pants is a disaster on a pear-shaped body with a long waist for the Sporty Style Statement. The light color and side pockets add weight to full hips, and the cropped-length makes your legs look shorter and take your body further out of balance. However, inverted triangles, rectangles and the hourglass shape can embrace them. This is a category where every purchase should be carefully considered to ensure it suits your body shape to fit and flatter.

When buying skirts, the length is critical for women over 40. There are many great options, but they are narrowed with each passing year. Wearing a skirt too short can make you appear that you are dressing too young, which actually makes you look older; and a long, full skirt, to the ankle, can be too dowdy.

There are three skirt lengths that flatter most women: a few inches above the knee (for women who are in great shape with beautiful legs), mid-length at the knee and the just below the calf muscle. Avoid having a skirt fall at the thickest part of the calf—in the middle of your calf muscle—it will make the legs look shorter and wider. One exception is a long, slim skirt that falls to the floor; it can look elegant and elongate your body when worn correctly, based on your body shape.

Dresses are challenging for women over 40; they feel so feminine and are pretty, but can be fraught with fit issues from top to bottom. Additionally, so many dresses at retail stores are sleeveless or bare. If you find a dress you love and don't feel comfortable baring your arms, a shrug or wide scarf can come in handy to keep you feeling more confident.

When considering a dress, the first rule is to wear proper under-garments—a bra with great support and a shaper may be necessary, depending on the fabric and style. Dresses can be versatile and changed easily by adding a cardigan, jacket or belt. They can be more forgiving to the body shape, and can be more flattering due to the primarily solid or single swath of fabric that extends down your body to lengthen you.

Jeans
__2 Basic __2 Trendy
__1 Trouser Style

Slacks
__2 Black __1 Mid-Tone
__1 Light Color

Skirts
Casual/Weekend
__1 Slim __1 Fashion

Dressy/Career
__1 Slim __1 Fashion

Dresses
Casual/Weekend
__1 Black __1 Color

Dressy/Career
__1 Black __1 Color

Formal/Evening
__1 Black __1 Color

THE ACCENT WARDROBE

Accent pieces are fun! They allow you to make a unique style expression. They can become a signature look, conversation starter or create a memorable Style Statement. This is where you can really enjoy expressing yourself.

Accent pieces are head-to-toe accessory items that include jewelry, scarves, belts, shoes and purses. Style takes on a more interesting, modern and individualized approach when these pieces are coordinated rather than matched.

Accent pieces create a finished look to an outfit. A generous assortment of options helps add more creativity and variety to your look. However, the same body shape rules apply to accessories as when you are choosing garments. For instance, if you are selecting a belt and you have a short waist, it would be best to avoid wide styles.

Jewelry
__1 Watch   __3 Earrings   __3 Necklaces

Scarves
__1 Black   __2 Colors

Purses

Dressy/Career   Casual/Weekend
__1 Black __1 Brown   __1 Black __1 Neutral

Formal/Evening
__1 Black __1 Metallic

Shoes

Closed Toe
__1 Black __1 Brown __1 Neutral

Open Toe
__1 Black __1 Brown __1 Neutral

Casual Sandals
__1 Black __1 Brown __1 Neutral

Boots
__1 Tall __1 Ankle __1 Neutral

Tennis Shoes
___1 White

Belts

Thin
__1 Black ___1 Brown __1 Metallic

Wide
__1 Black __1 Brown

You've done all the work—examining, preparing and planning—now it's time to go shopping! The next step arms you with the best shopping skills to maximize your time.

Step 7:

SHOPPING WITH A PLAN

Shopping often begins with enthusiasm, anticipating the excitement of bringing home new clothes that make you feel pretty. Unfortunately, the excitement can quickly dim after a few trips to the fitting room and end with your self-confidence taking a dive. It's no wonder many women over 40 say, "I hate to shop, but I still love to look great."

The three shopping strategies below can help you prevent shopping frustration, and increase the odds of having a successful and pleasant shopping experience. By starting with a plan and following some of the "tricks of the trade" used by fashion designers and stylists, shopping can become an enjoyable experience with an exciting outcome. You can shop like a pro and feel like a million by the end of your shopping trip.

PLANNING

Set a shopping goal: Determine what you want or need and plan to spend your time focused on your goal—do not deviate.

Review magazines for ideas: This is a great way to expand your view and give you ideas that you may have never thought of before. Look at a variety of magazines to help expand your thoughts (a new accessory or how to wear it, a new color, etc.). Tear out pages of styles that appeal to you. When you have looked through each magazine, review the pages you tore out and prioritize them by your favorite choices.

Plan where you will shop: Take a look at your favorite clothing items, and then look at the brands of each item and the stores where you bought them. These details can give you a clue about what works best—these are most likely the brands/stores that cater to you. Begin by making a list of the items and the brands/stores. This will give you an idea of where to start to get the best possible shopping outcome. Branch out from there by going online and doing a search for those brands/stores. See what other brands/stores come up in the search—those might also be good for you to consider. You can also think about trying new shopping centers you have not visited in awhile or have always wanted to try.

Create a shopping list: Work from your **Balanced Wardrobe List** and write the details of the items you want and where you plan to find them. Prioritize your list and stick to it. Make this your roadmap that you will follow for the day.

Make a pact with yourself to stay focused: Once you arrive, there are so many temptations along the way that will attract

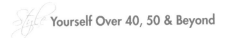

your attention, especially if you haven't been shopping in awhile. If you want to explore those items that caught your eye but are not on your list, make a note of them and go back after you have completed your priorities for the day.

Clear your calendar of obligations: Make sure you have set aside enough uninterrupted time to complete your shopping. As we all know, we don't get out and shop as often as we need or like; so make sure that when you do, you make it count. If your phone rings, unless you must, let it go to voicemail or text back if necessary. This is your time, protect it; you are doing something special for yourself.

SHOPPING

Shop alone: Shopping alone will keep you focused and allow you to control your schedule. You will not feel obligated to be mindful of anyone else's time or schedule, and you can indulge in this time spent just for you. Also, you will not be influenced by someone else's idea of what you should have or how you should look.

Dress in simple pieces that are easy to remove: Your incentive to try on clothes will be stronger if you are wearing clothing that is easy to take off. It is best to take a layer of clothing, a sweater or jacket if the weather changes. You can keep it in the car until you need an extra layer of warmth.

Wear a small amount of makeup: It is a good idea to wear just enough makeup to feel pretty, but a small amount that can give you the confidence that you will not rub makeup off on clothing you try on. You will also find that customer service will be better when you are seen as a fashionable, serious shopper. When you are ready for their help, salespeople will be more eager to help you find the sizes or styles you need.

Bring energy bars: Shopping can be a physical task and it is important to keep your energy high until you are finished. To stay focused and efficient with your time, it is helpful to have an energy bar handy when you feel hungry rather than spending time looking for a place to eat.

Replace a large purse with a small shopping purse: You will be so grateful by the end of the day that you followed this advice. Your purse may feel manageable at the start of your trip but, after a few hours, the weight of a filled purse will feel intolerable on your shoulders and your back. The best idea is to find a small shoulder purse to stash the bare essentials such as your keys, wallet, cell phone, small digital camera, notepad and energy bar.

Wear time-tested comfortable shoes: This is not a time to wear shoes just for style; we are going for comfort here. The goal is to leave the end of your shopping day with all the items on your list that you love with minimal wear on your feet.

Bring quarters for street meters: Parking will be easier, faster and more convenient if you bring quarters. They will expand your parking options if you are visiting a store with limited parking accommodations, or you may want to quickly check out a store that caught your eye from the street. While many meters have been updated to accept credit cards, many still have not. It's best to be prepared. This will ensure you will never have to waste time by searching for someone to give you change or not be able to visit a store because you couldn't find parking nearby.

EVALUATING

Select items that reflect your Style Statement and personality: Evaluate each item you are considering with the same criteria you used when you cleaned your closet. Critique the item to make sure it reflects your Style Statement, works for your body shape and has the most flattering fit with quality fabric.

As designers and stylists, we are always shopping with a very specific personality and Style Statement of a customer in mind. Before we begin shopping, we have complete clarity about our customer's profile and Style Statement needs. This helps us have the best possible outcome for a successful shopping trip to ensure our customers are happy. The same is true when you shop for yourself. Get clear about your needs and your style before you shop. Take your lists with you if you to staff focused and organized. You are the stylist and you are shopping for your best customer: You!

Make peace with your current body shape: Although you may have plans to lose weight, it will work against you if you are judging your body by how you want to look versus how you look now. You will feel so much better when you find something that flatters you and that you can wear today. Make sure you only buy items you can wear proudly now, not when you lose a specified amount of weight as a "goal" item to give you the incentive to lose weight. Chances are you will feel so much better about yourself if you find an amazing outfit that makes you look 10 pounds lighter . . . instantly!

Don't buy anything you don't love: Do not compromise. If you don't love it and are trying to talk yourself into buying something, it means you have not found the perfect item—keep shopping. Make sure you always look in a three-way mirror to see the item you are considering and how it looks from all angles, especially from the back. Resist the temptation to look at price tags. In the long run, you will spend far less money buying the few things you love, that make you feel beautiful, than many items that you don't wear very often and don't make you feel good about yourself.

Bring a camera: You may find a few styles that you like and are having a tough time making a decision. Or, you may find something you like but want to wait before making a decision. A camera is a handy resource to store ideas and give you quick recall for later. If you don't have a camera, you can use a notebook.

Part 4:

THE FINAL TOUCH

Defining details that
make a big difference

As you have focused your time, money and attention on updating your wardrobe, the finishing touches need special attention, too. If neglected, they can diminish all the hard work you have put into your overall appearance.

Step 1: Assessing the State of Your Beauty Maintenance Needs

Step 2: Maintaining Your Crowning Jewel

Step 3: Putting Your Best Face Forward

Step 4: Pampering Your Polished Accent

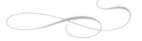

Step 1:

ASSESSING THE STATE OF YOUR BEAUTY MAINTENANCE NEEDS

The finishing touches—hair, your crowning jewel; make-up, your best face forward; nails, your polished accent— are the important embellishments to communicate your Identity and Image. By giving attention to these details, it will help you look better, feel better about yourself and signal to the world that you lovingly take care and pride in your self-care.

If you have not consistently maintained your beauty routine, it may seem overwhelming at first. But, you don't need to do it all at once. The best place to start is with the area you think needs your attention the most. Once you begin, you will see how much fun it is and that will help move you confidently forward to other areas.

For women over 40, in earlier years, some of the time required for beauty was minimal or you could get by with a simple do-it-yourself maintenance routine. While you still may be able to keep a few DIY tasks intact, this is the time in life to consider raising your beauty game by outsourcing the help of qualified professional specialists, otherwise known as your personal Glam Squad—they can give you guided instruction for top-notch care.

Determining how many members you will need on your Glam Squad and how often you will see them depends on the demands of your Lifestyle and the urgency of your beauty issues. For instance, if you have a Lifestyle where you stay at home, you will have different needs than if you are a Socializer with a heavy business networking schedule.

But first, how do you know which area of your style needs the most attention or if you are even out of style? Maybe there is something about your style that has been bothering you. If you made the change in this one area and it would make you feel much better, that would be the place to start. If you are still not sure where to start, you can think about asking for feedback from a trusted friend with a sense of style you admire. You could approach it as an open-ended question or ask for an opinion about how they would prioritize the three areas you are considering changing.

The **Finishing Touch Assessment Guide** below can serve as a visual guide to see the state of your beauty maintenance needs. Once you have completed it, you will be guided towards the areas that may need the most attention.

When you truly recognize the power of updating and keeping your finishing touches at their best, you will make the investment in your time and money and raise your beauty game. By valuing these beauty assets, you will spend the time on yourself, and it will dra-

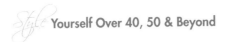

matically change your overall look and how you feel. I can't state this enough. No matter what state of mind you are in about your body, and I hope it is positive, but if not, tending to your finishing touches will make you feel better yourself overall. It can serve as a nice confidence booster. Just think about how you feel when you leave a salon after a flattering haircut. You may feel that you want to get your car washed, straighten your bedroom, put on a little lip gloss . . . you get the idea . . . attending to one area creates a spillover effect into other areas of self-care, and the overall effect is beneficial to your looks and your life.

Finishing Touch Assessment Guide

On a scale of 1 to 10, with 1 being the lowest level of care and 10 the highest, circle the number that best represents your level of care within each area.

Hair
Style   1   2   3   4   5   6   7   8   9   10

Hair Color
Base color   1   2   3   4   5   6   7   8   9   10
Gray coverage 1   2   3   4   5   6   7   8   9   10

Skin
Complexion quality 1   2   3   4   5   6   7   8   9   10

Makeup
Foundation   1   2   3   4   5   6   7   8   9   10
Eyes   1   2   3   4   5   6   7   8   9   10
Lips   1   2   3   4   5   6   7   8   9   10

Nails

Fingernails	1	2	3	4	5	6	7	8	9	10
Cuticles	1	2	3	4	5	6	7	8	9	10

Feet

Toenails	1	2	3	4	5	6	7	8	9	10
Dry heels	1	2	3	4	5	6	7	8	9	10

If you rated yourself a 3 or below, this is an area that needs prompt attention and is best served by a professional.

Step 2:

MAINTAINING YOUR CROWNING JEWEL

HAIR COLOR

As we age, there are a variety of changes we will experience with our hair, and gray hair is the first indication we are aging. Your hair may turn partially or all gray, become thin, change texture or lose luster. These changes will affect your color, styling choices and options.

The age when your hair begins to turn gray, and how much gray hair you will ultimately have, is determined by genetics. Some women make a choice to wear their hair all gray while others prefer to color. Whatever choice you make, there should be no middle ground. Loose gray strands of hair create a perception of lackluster self-care and do not present a polished image.

If you choose to go all gray, it requires that all other areas of your style be impeccably maintained for an updated look; otherwise, you could run the risk of going "Granny." The cut should be modern, well styled with equally modern makeup and clothing. The image of Meryl Streep in *The Devil Wears Prada* is at the highest level of head-to-toe maintenance and taste for going gray the right way. However, there are many beautiful examples of wearing gray with style; but, the big message is, "If you do it, go all the way . . . your way!"

If gray hair does not flatter you, and you are not doing the required maintenance to keep it free from stray gray hairs, it is time to look into the reasons you are not taking care of yourself. If it is a time issue, it may be helpful for you to regularly schedule hair color appointments on your calendar in advance for an entire year. You can estimate the time frame when gray strands begin to show, which is usually from six to eight weeks for most women. This will ensure you will always step out looking your best.

Selecting the right shade to color your hair is an important step. It can be a wise investment to visit a professional colorist who can guide you towards your best color choices. The colors that complemented you in your 20s and 30s may not work as well over 40. Changes in your complexion and facial structure can affect the tones and shades that can age you or make you appear years younger. You can visit a salon for a consultation then match the color from a home option.

If money is keeping you from staying on top of your hair color routine, there are excellent home color products. This is also a great option if time and money are keeping you from maintaining your hair color. The only exception to coloring your hair yourself is if you are planning to go several shades lighter. In this case, it is best to work with a professional colorist to avoid the risk of damaging your hair, and to make sure you get the desired result.

My favorite home hair coloring products:

Clairol Gray Solution

When stray grays appear, keep this product near! Apply color; wait 20 minutes . . . gray is gone. Usually lasts from four to six weeks.

- Complete gray coverage

- Easy to use

- Large color selection

Clairol Perfect 10

When you want to quickly remove gray hair, this will take care of it in 10 minutes, and it works.

- Fast and easy

- Inexpensive

HAIR STYLE

When updating, the fastest way to a modern look is with a new haircut. Sometimes just a trim can make a difference by helping your hair to look healthier by removing split ends and adding shape. When making an appointment with a stylist, request a consultation with the colorist to give you advice after your new cut.

There are really no rules when it comes to hairstyle, length and age. The only rule is to choose a style you love that looks great on you. The best guidance is to consider the texture, your face shape and your Style Statement. The quality of your hair can change with age, becoming brittle or thin, especially during menopause when the production of keratin slows the rate of growth. The hair strands become thin, fine and lose pigment, so it becomes lighter in color. Some hair follicles stop producing hair altogether.

Some women find that their smooth hair of younger years has become coarse and dry. Others have the opposite experience with hair that was once coarse has become thin and limp. The hairstyles that worked before need fresh new options to work with the new texture.

If your formerly coarse hair has turned thin and limp, adding volume back to the hair shaft is the goal. For styling options, the ideal length is to keep it at shoulder length or above. Side swept bangs work easily with thin, fine hair. They look stylish, frame your face and add a youthful lift. Resist using straightening tools and trade for hot rollers to add lift and body. Combined with a volumizing spray, it can give your hair a fuller, thicker appearance.

If your formerly smooth hair has turned coarse and dry, reducing bulk and weight is the goal. By cutting layers into your hair, it will allow your hair to look lighter, feel lighter and add movement. This will also make your hair easier to manage. Coarse hair needs moisture and shine to keep it looking its best. Deep conditioning treatments will give back the needed moisture, and adding a serum on towel-dried hair prior to blow drying will give it shine.

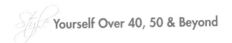
Considering Your Face Shape

Choosing a hairstyle that is perfect for your face shape will enhance your best features. There are several different approaches to determining your face shape. However, I find that most of them are complicated and create more questions than answers. So after contemplating the various ways, I decided to share with you the way I think is the simplest.

How to Measure:

You'll need a mirror, measuring tape and your best judgment.

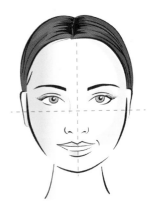

Stand in front of the mirror and take "flat" measurements (take straight down/side-to-side measurements).

Face Length: Measure in a straight line from the top of your forehead to the tip of your chin.

Face Width: Begin by placing the tape measure at your cheekbone on one side of your face, at the hairline. Measure horizontally, across the bridge of your nose to the other side of your face.

My face length is: _____

My face width is: _____

Now, take a look at your measurements and determine (using your best judgment) which of the following seven face shapes most closely resembles your face.

OVAL

The length of your face is 1.5 times the width

Best Styles: All hair lengths, hair off your face

Styles to Avoid: Heavy bangs, hair in your face

Oval Celebrities: Cindy Crawford, Julia Roberts, Courtney Cox, Sharon Stone

ROUND

The length of your face is equal to the width

Best Styles: Fullness at the crown, side parts, side bangs, face-framing layers

Styles to Avoid: Chin length, center parts, straight bangs, fullness at the side of the face

Round Celebrities: Kate Winslet, Ingrid Bergman, Drew Barrymore

RECTANGLE

The length of your face is longer than the width

Best Styles: Short or medium length, layers and fullness, side and center parts

Styles to Avoid: Long length, straight styles

Rectangle Celebrities: Kirstie Alley, Janet Jackson, Nicki Taylor, SJP

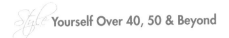

SQUARE

The length of your face is equal to the width, but more angular than a round face

Best Styles: Short to medium length, bangs and wispy layers, height at the crown

Styles to Avoid: Accentuating styles—long straight styles, straight bangs, center parts, bob ending at the jaw

Square Celebrities: Demi Moore, Isabella Roselini

HEART

Your jaw narrows in comparison to your forehead and cheekbones

Best Styles: Chin-length bobs, side parts, side bangs, layers around the face

Styles to Avoid: Short and full styles, height at the crown, full bangs, hair off the forehead

Heart Celebrities: Jennifer Love Hewitt, Naomi Campbell, Michelle Pfeiffer

DIAMOND

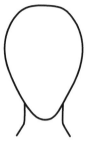

Your forehead and jaw are narrow in comparison to your cheekbones

Best Styles: Hair off your face, all hair lengths, narrow at the sides, fullness at the crown

Styles to Avoid: Hair in your face

Diamond Celebrities: Linda Evangelista, Sophia Loren, Nicole Kidman

TRIANGLE

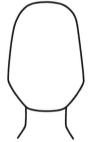

Your jaw is your widest measurement; your cheeks and forehead get smaller

Best Styles: Short hair, fullness at the crown, full at forehead, narrow at the chin, side parts, layers

Styles to Avoid: Full styles, long length, center parts, height at the crown

Triangle Celebrities: Kathy Ireland, Victoria Beckham

My face shape is: _____

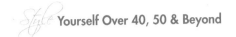

Considering Your Lifestyle and Style Statement

The best approach when choosing a style is one that is based on your Lifestyle *and* your Style Statement. This will ensure you will consistently maintain the upkeep of your hair *and* achieve an overall balanced appearance. By choosing a style based on your Lifestyle, you take into consideration how you spend most of your time. This practical approach asks that you realistically take into account the demands of your daily life. You will then be able to make the most accurate decision about how much time you have and are willing to devote to grooming your hair.

The next step in selecting your hairstyle is to take your Style Statement into consideration. Take a close look at the traits and attributes for your Style Statement. Think about how these descriptive adjectives could look when translated to a hairstyle. Take your time and look through magazines or search online to find different styles that appeal to you. Narrow the styles down by looking at them and layering the words to the styles that most closely bring these words to life. This approach will help connect your hair to your Style Statement clothing choices for an overall seamless and stunning authentic style.

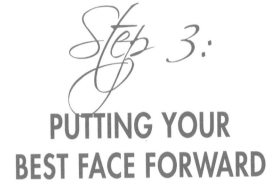

PUTTING YOUR
BEST FACE FORWARD

Our skin changes over 40 and there are a variety of issues we may be managing due to fluctuating hormones. Before there is a focus on makeup, the priority should be the quality of your skin. Your beautiful face is one of the most important first impressions you will make as you meet people and look into their eyes. Make the most of it by using the right products for your skin, the right colors for your tone, and modern application techniques to maximize your beauty and prevent adding years to your face. It is easy to get into a makeup rut and look dated, since trends change and evolve over the years.

The tone and texture of our skin changes with age, and the products you use need to change with it. As we age, our skin produces less melanin—the pigment that allows skin to tan instead of burn. A reduction in melanin decreases your skin's natural ability to protect you from the sun's harmful UV rays. This is why it is more important than ever to protect your skin from the sun. The first line of defense to keep skin looking beautiful is to increase your sun protection by using a high quality block that will give you total protection.

After 40, our skin needs a different level of care with products that counter the effects of aging, especially moisture loss. We produce new skin cells at a slower rate and oil glands become enlarged. When skin does not exfoliate as fast, it leaves behind dead skin cells that can clog pores and create acne. That's why a gentle and effective cleansing routine that includes exfoliation becomes more important than ever.

My favorite sunscreen: Cotz Total Block. I feel completely protected from the sun's aging rays when I wear this incredible sunscreen. It's my anti-aging beauty secret; I won't leave the house without it.

- Keeps skin protected to stay young looking, free from fine lines and brown spots

- Will not clog pores or cause breakouts

- Wear alone or under foundation

My favorite skin cleanser: Magic Mitt. My number one all-star favorite product to keep my skin clean and clear! It amazes me every time I use it!

- Cleans and exfoliates without cleanser

- Reusable and durable

- Easily removes all makeup, even mascara!

As we age, skin loses natural moisture because fluctuating hormones are less effective at stimulating oil glands. Without consistently functioning oil glands, skin can become dry, itchy or flakey. Combined with a reduction in collagen production, skin gets thinner, loses firmness and begins to show more fine lines. Adding moisture back into the skin with the right moisturizer is a critical step in the over 40 beauty routine.

My favorite moisturizers: Egyptian Magic and **Shea Butter 100% Pure Face Cream by Now**. These moisturizes are simple, safe and effective. The older I get, the more simplicity I crave in my skin care routine. Also, my skin has become more sensitive; I can treat it gently and keep it looking its best with these products of perfection!

- Maintains skin's moisture balance and evens skin tone

- Will not clog pores or cause breakouts; chemical free

My favorite acne fighter: Mario Badesco Drying Lotion. Adult acne is so annoying, but I've got something formidable to fight back. This is a little pink acne-fighting miracle in a bottle. Just place a dab on the pimple, let dry and keep on overnight . . . be prepared to be amazed!

- Dries quickly

- Eliminates breakouts overnight

UPDATING WITH MAKEUP

Some product lines are especially formulated for mature skin and can make you look years younger! If you have not changed the way you apply makeup or you have been using the same brand for ten or more years, it's time to get acquainted with new lines and updated with a makeup lesson. My philosophy about makeup is to take your time to find the highest quality products that work the most effectively for you. I don't believe in skimping on products you use on your face. I'd rather buy fewer high quality products than many products at a lower quality. I have found that the right products really make a difference to give a polished, finished look.

The most effective approach to applying makeup over 40 is the combination of selecting products that are specially formulated for your skin and age, making an investment in the proper tools, and mastering application skills.

Beauty Blunders That Can Add Years To Your Face

Skin:

- Foundation that is applied too heavily

- Foundation that is improperly color matched

- Foundation that has not been blended properly

- Setting powders or mineral makeup powders that settle into fine lines

- Heavy blush on cheeks

Eyes:

- Shiny eye shadow

- Colorful or bright eye shadow

- Heavy mascara on upper and lower lashes

- Black eyeliner or applied with a heavy, thick line

- Under-eye concealer not blended completely or a shade too light

- Thin eyebrows that have been overly plucked

Lips:

- Over-plumped cosmetic lip procedure

- Visible lip liner

- Lip color that is too dark

There are so many ways to get and stay updated with makeup. Sephora carries most lines and their qualified beauty experts are eager to patiently spend time with you to find the best product match and give you detailed application instruction. Department store counters are also an option. Merle Norman makeup studios also offer free makeovers with no obligation to buy products.

One of the best ways to avoid beauty blunders—once you have all the right tools and you are ready to apply your makeup with skillful application—is to make sure you can see yourself clearly! If you don't already have one, this may be the time to invest in a magnifying makeup mirror with bright lighting.

My favorite lighted makeup mirror: Jerdon Lighted Makeup Mirror. This mirror saves me from leaving the house with crooked eyeliner and/or applying too much makeup. A beauty lifesaver!

- Magnified close-up mirror view allows you to apply makeup more precisely

- Manage your beauty maintenance routine more accurately

Product And Application Guidelines To Putting Your Best Face Forward Over 40

Foundation

As our skin ages, it loses moisture, and the best foundations are those that replace needed moisture with hydration. If you need more coverage, these can be layered just on the areas of your face where you need it most. Some foundations are specifically formulated for mature skin and have light-reflecting pigments to deflect the look of wrinkles, antioxidants to keep skin healthy and moisture to keep skin supple looking. Always use high quality makeup sponges or brushes to apply foundation. Avoid using matte or powder foundations that can emphasize wrinkles.

Pay close attention to the color of your foundation to make sure you get the right match. It's always a good idea to apply a sample of the foundation and look at it indoors and outdoors before you buy. Steer clear of any products that contain bismuth oxide or oxychloride. It is used by many cosmetic companies, primarily in mineral makeup as a filler ingredient to keep it from sliding off your face. Therefore, the foundation seeps more deeply into your pores and can trigger a variety of allergic reactions such as redness, inflammation, cause cystic acne and make rosacea flare up. Please, read your labels!

My favorite foundation: Silk Crème Foundation by Laura Mercier. Specially formulated for mature skin, this oil-free foundation has light-reflecting qualities that minimize fine lines, perfect for aging skin! The creamy consistency glides on and evens out skin tone—love it!

- Made with black tea extracts for skin friendly antioxidant benefits

- Can be layered in target areas to double as a cover-up

My favorite setting powder: Make Up For Ever HD Micro-finish Powder. This amazing powder gives a flawless, polished finish to your face. Definitely gives the extra "wow" factor, and the only powder I'll use on my over 40 face!

- Creates a smooth, flawless looking complexion

- Specially formulated for mature skin, smoothes fine lines and imperfections

- Eliminates shine and can be used alone or over foundation

My favorite makeup sponges: Makeup Sponges by Laura Mercier. These high quality sponges provide complete control when applying foundation for a smooth, even and streak-free application every time. They are so durable, I've had mine for over a decade and they still look and perform like new!

- Oval shape maneuvers easily around contours of face

- Antibacterial

- Soft, perfect for sensitive skin

My favorite makeup brushes: Sephora Makeup Brushes. They have one of the most comprehensive selections of brushes you will find. There's a brush for every makeup application.

- Excellent selection

- Unbeatable value for the level of quality

- Patient and knowledgeable staff to help you make the right selection

Eye Makeup

The windows to your soul are your strongest focal point. The delicate, thin skin around your eyes is one of the first areas of the face to develop fine lines and show signs of aging. As gravity takes hold, the eyes lose lid space and definition. Makeup can bring focus back to the eyes; however, the colors, brands and application techniques will need to change with the changes of the skin quality and aging of your eyes.

Brows

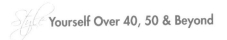

Thick brows are a sign of health and youth. As we age, we lose hair all over our entire bodies, including our brows. Also the brows get lighter on some women. It is common to lose the outside third of brows or they can become thin from years over plucking, giving the appearance of looking older. Additionally, plucking can cause damage to the hair shaft and inflame the hair follicles. This causes hair to grow back finer and shorter. Over time, hair follicles shrink and produce skinnier, shorter strands, then die off and never grow back.

If your brows have become thin from hair loss or are victims of over plucking, there's help. Hide your tweezers and don't pluck for three months. This will give your hair follicles a chance to heal and recover to prepare for regrowth. As some of the hair grows back, you'll begin to see your natural arch and can resume plucking stray strands. However, make sure you use high quality tweezers to prevent breakage and continued damage. Additionally, you can fill in the sparse areas of your brows with a brow pencil. It is important to buy a high quality pencil to create the finest line strokes for a more natural appearance. Otherwise, you could end up with dark, drawn in looking brows that will be even more aging than skinny brows.

My favorite brow filler: Anastasia Brow Wiz. The most natural looking, easy-to-apply brow enhancer . . . it's my favorite! Defined brows add strength and focus to eyes for dramatic impact.

- Lifts the eyes for younger looking, thicker brows

- Retractable, never needs sharpening

- Super-fine tip creates more natural looking brows

My favorite tweezers: Slant-Tip Expert Tweezers by

Revlon. I have bought the best, high-end tweezers and spent so much more. For performance and durability, you can't beat these!

- Angled tip

- Perfect alignment and tension

- Non-slip to hold with ease

Eye Shadow

There are a variety of age-related changes to adjust to with eyes. From loose skin on the lid to gravity causing eyes to appear droopy, the right application and color choices can go a long way towards bringing back a vibrant, alert look. Light colors applied right below the brow bone, with medium color shades on the crease extending to the outer side of the eyelid, will make eyes appear larger and less droopy, and will give them a lift. Darker colors close the eye, making eyes look smaller and giving them a sleepy appearance, and should be avoided.

A lid primer is essential before applying eye shadow on over 40 lids. It will prevent the eye shadow from sliding into the creases of your eyelids and keep the makeup in place to look freshly applied all day long. Invest in a few good brushes for application and blending. It will help make your application faster, easier, more precise and professional looking.

My favorite eye shadow primer: Shadow Insurance by Too Faced. This primer keeps color in place and helps it blend better. I won't wear eye shadow without it!

- Smoothes lines on lids for more even coverage

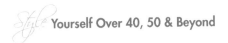

- Highly concentrated formula, a little drop covers the entire lid

My favorite eye shadow: Laura Mercier Eye Shadow. It glides on to create a long-wearing and crease resistant finish perfect for over 40 lids!

- Formulated for mature skin

- Creamy matte formula

- Huge color selection

Eyeliner

Eyeliner can become one of the most frustrating makeup moments to remind you of your age. There will come a time, if it has not already happened—or, if you can remember when it happened—when the skin on your eyelids will move when you apply eyeliner. The same liner that may have worked perfectly for years, one day, just won't create a smooth, single line when you move it across your lid. It tugs, and you have to go back and fill in. Welcome to your middle-age moment.

The first step is to use a liner with a softer formula, one that will glide on easily. The next application technique is to gently pull your eyelid towards your ear to stretch it out. While stretching, apply the eyeliner with your other hand.

Finally, the choice of eyeliner color may need to change, too. The dark eyeliners that have always worked so well are not flattering to women as we age. It will close the eyes and give you the appearance of looking sleepy, or older. A dark brown or eggplant color will be softer and add depth to your eye.

My favorite eyeliner: Quickliner for Eyes by Clinique.
Gone are the days where creepy lids cause the liner to skip. This
creamy formula goes on smooth and stays put all day.

- 3-in-1 with liner, smudger and eye shadow

- Retractable, never needs sharpening

Mascara

**As we age, our lashes may need extra help to look as full as
they once did in our younger years.** They become thinner, brittle and break more easily. When lashes fall out, they are replaced at
a slower rate with finer, shorter lashes. But the chemicals in mascara
can contribute to breakage. Plus, layers of mascara are also difficult
to remove completely without excessive rubbing. That can accelerate
the loss of lashes. It's a viscous cycle . . . putting mascara on to make
lashes appear longer and thicker . . . losing lashes . . . putting mascara on to make them appear longer and thicker . . . losing lashes . . .

The best way to apply mascara to thin lashes is to start at the base
and move the brush sideways, and then outward. Applying a thicker
layer near the outer edge of the eyelids make eyelashes look thicker
and eyes larger. A lash curler will curl lashes to open your eyes and
make them sparkle.

My favorite mascara: Lash Blast Mascara by Covergirl.
This drugstore delivers luxury brand results! Get long, thick and
curly lashes with just a few strokes.

- Unbeatable price and value to rival much higher priced brands

- Lengthens, thickens and curls lashes

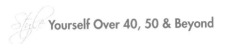

My favorite eyelash curler: She Uemura Eyelash Curler.
This eyelash curler didn't get its iconic status without earning it.
You'll love how easily it curls without pinching or pulling your eyelids.

- Creates smooth, long lasting curl

- Safely curls lashes with the perfect amount of pressure from the patented hinge technology

My favorite false eyelashes: Ardell Accents Lashes, Style #301. If you need a little extra assist, these are the most natural and easiest to apply lashes I have used. They are strip lashes and only for the outer corners of the eye.

- Durable and reusable

- Natural looking; made from 100% human hair

- So easy to apply!

Lips

Lips start to become dry and require more conditioning and care than ever before. Exposure to the sun and outdoor elements, combined with the natural aging process, reduce moisture. Additionally, they can lose some color, shape and fullness through the years. Fortunately, there are great options to keep them looking soft and kissable.

By exfoliating lips, it can go a long way towards making them a soft and smooth palette before applying color. Moisturizing lips with a lip gloss or balm plumps them up making them appear more youthful and healthy. A lip primer can define lips and help avoid feathering with your lip color. You can also use a lip liner to keep lipstick in place. A flesh-colored lip pencil is a great option as a versatile primer.

Many glosses are too shiny and sticky or they don't last all day. Lipstick formulas can be too thick and drying or too formal for a daytime look. The alternative is to team a gloss layered over your lipstick color. The shine will give your lips a fuller, pouter, sexier look.

My favorite lip product: Lip Smoothie by Clinique. Formulated for mature lips, it's vitamin-fortified to add moisture, fullness and reduce the appearance of fine lines, all while looking gorgeous!

- The perfect hybrid of a gloss and lipstick

- Just the right amount of age-appropriate shine

- Great to wear alone or layer over lipstick to soften

Step 4:

PAMPERING YOUR
POLISHED ACCENT

Caring for your nails is an important part of maintaining beautiful, fashionable, well-groomed hands and feet. In addition to being a symbol of creativity and beauty, they are also a reflection of your health. Your nails change with age. Since hair and nails both contain protein, they undergo similar changes. They grow more slowly and can become dull and brittle. They can even change color by becoming yellow and opaque. Sometimes ridges can develop. By following a simple beauty routine, you can keep hands and nails beautiful for life.

The sun is the cause of 90 percent to 95 percent of wrinkles, lines and discolorations to our bodies and hands. By keeping sunblock in your car and applying it to the back of your hands, it can help reduce sun damage that causes sunspots and dryness.

By moisturizing the nails and cuticles, it will keep skin smooth and supple. Natural fingernails in a short to medium length with a round or square shape will keep hands youthful looking. The choice of colors can range from natural to fashion shades.

My favorite nail polish: Orly Nail Polish. This is the most long-lasting nail polish I have used, and they have a stunningly beautiful selection of colors. The formula gives you salon quality nails at home.

- Excellent quality to rival salon brands

- Long-lasting formula and fast drying time

- Free from DBP, toluene, formaldehyde and resin

Part 5:

MAINTAIN YOUR AUTHENTIC STYLE

Staying modern for a lifetime

Just as important as it was for you to make changes to your style from the inside out, it is equally as important to maintain your beautiful results. The final part of your program has three steps to help you continue the commitment you have made to yourself. By having these tools in place, they will keep you focused and inspired.

Step 1: Stay Flawless for a Lifetime with "The 10 Commitments of Style"

Step 2: Your Unique Style Profile at a Glance

Step 3: Maintaining Your Balanced Wardrobe

Step 1:

STAY FLAWLESS FOR A LIFETIME WITH "THE 10 COMMITMENTS OF STYLE"

You have updated your style so beautifully and authentically—it will serve you well for years to come. However, there may be times when you need an extra boost of style motivation. So, the first step is to make a commitment to maintaining all of the hard work you have achieved so far.

The following contract is a sacred style pact you are making with yourself. By signing and dating it, you are making a loving commitment to practice self-care and honor all that is unique about you and the courage to express it to the world!

Once you have read it, please sign and date it only when you feel ready to make the commitment. When you are ready, tear it out or make a copy and place it in your closet. By keeping this contract visible, the 10 Commitments will be reinforced and eventually ingrained in the way you treat yourself for a lifetime!

My Style Contract:
The 10 Commitments

On this day _____, **I am making a commitment to love myself and reflect it to the world through my style. I will consistently follow these rules to maintain my uniquely modern and hip style over 40.**

1. I will make thoughtful and strategic Style Statement purchases.

2. I will express my authentic Style Statement in every purchase.

3. I will only buy what I love—items that make me look and feel beautiful.

4. I will dress for my horizontal and vertical body shape.

5. I will keep and maintain a Balanced Wardrobe List in my closet.

6. I will plan and prepare before I shop.

7. I will give up buying aspirational clothing to use as weight-loss incentives.

8. I will maintain an organized closet.

9. I will give up the need to try on only one size when I shop.

10. I will love and accept myself for who I am today, not for who I was or who I want to be.

Signed _____

Step 2:

YOUR UNIQUE STYLE PROFILE AT A GLANCE

This step is a critically important part of the final work we will be doing together. This is really the heart of the program, the part where we see the essence of who you are and how it translates to your Signature Style. I think it's so exciting when you can see it all come together in one area. It's like having a very special mirror held up for you with a comprehensive, 360-degree view.

For you to have a complete view, you will need to fill in all the spaces. This is a compilation of your Unique Style Profile. It combines every aspect of all the things that make you the beautiful person you are. It serves as a snapshot to remind you of how you will be expressing yourself on the outside to stay true to your personal Style Statement.

Once you have completed this step, you can either tear it out to make a mini-booklet of your Unique Style Profile to be kept as a reference for quick review when needed or you can keep it here in the book for easy access.

You may also find that as you move throughout different transitions in your journey of life over 40, as your lifestyle changes, your style needs will change. You can refer back to the book and repeat the steps to update your Style Statement. This will help reflect the practical needs of your new lifestyle. You can use this book to maintain your style for life!

MY UNIQUE STYLE PROFILE

Identity and Image (page 29)

Primary Identity _____

Primary Image _____

Secondary Identity _____

Secondary Image _____

Notes about my Identity and Image: _____

_____

_____

Style Statement (page 34)

My Style Statement is: _____

Notes about my Style Profile (Part 1, Step 5): _____

_____

_____

_____

Lifestyle (page 129)

My Lifestyle is: _____

Lifestyle Notes: _____

_____

_____

_____

_____

Body Shape

My Horizontal Body Shape is (page 66): _____

My Vertical Body Shape is (page 86): _____

Clothing Strategy Notes (Part 2, Steps 2 and 4):_____

_____

_____

_____

_____

_____

Colors (page 117)

Primary Color Palette

Color	Attributes	Effect

Secondary Color Palette

Color	Attributes	Effect

Notes about Color: _____

_____

_____

_____

_____

Hair Styles/Face Shape (page 161)

My face shape is: _____

Hairstyle Notes: _____

_____

_____

_____

_____

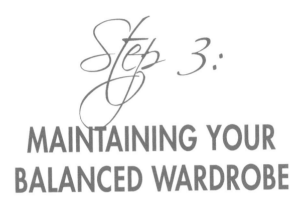

MAINTAINING YOUR BALANCED WARDROBE

Your Balanced Wardrobe List will allow you to maintain an organized, updated closet. You can refer to this handy list as often as needed. Some women find that using it monthly works for them, others seasonally, and some use it more often. However you choose to use it, the best way it will get used is to make sure it is visible.

By placing it in or around your closet, you can easily check the items that you need while it is fresh in your mind. This will create the list that forms the basis for strategic shopping; you will know exactly what you need.

When you are preparing to shop, review your Balanced Wardrobe List to make sure you prioritize the time you spend while you are out.

MY BALANCED WARDROBE LIST

Foundation Pieces

Undergarments
Bras

Seamless Push-Up
__2 Black __2 Nude

Strapless
__1 Nude

Racer Back
__1 Nude

Shapers

Midsection/Torso
__1 Nude

Hips and Thighs
__1 Nude

Tops
Camisoles
__1 black __1 White __Colors

Tank Tops
__1 Black __1 White __Colors

Short Sleeve T-Shirts
__1 Black __1 White

Long Sleeve T-Shirts
__1 Black __1 White

Pants
Lounge Pants
__1 Black __Colors

Notes:

_____

_____

_____

_____

_____

_____

_____

Statement Pieces

Tops

Short Sleeve T-Shirts

__3 Solid Colors

__1 Patterns/Prints

Long Sleeve T-Shirts

__3 Solid Colors

__1 Patterns/Prints

Shirts/Blouses

__3 Solid Colors __2 Patterns/Prints

Bottoms

Jeans

__2 Basic __2 Trendy

__1 Trouser Style

Slacks

__2 Black __1 Mid-Tone

__1 Light Color

Skirts

Casual/Weekend
__1 Slim __1 Fashion

Dressy/Career
__1 Slim __1 Fashion

Dresses

Casual/Weekend
__1 Black ___1 Color

Dressy/Career
__1 Black __1 Color

Formal/Evening
__1 Black __1 Color

Notes:

_____

_____

_____

_____

_____

_____

_____

Accent Pieces

Jewelry
__1 Watch   __3 Earrings   __3 Necklaces

Scarves
__1 Black   __2 Colors

Purses
Dressy/Career   Casual/Weekend
__1 Black __1 Brown   __1 Black __Neutral

Formal/Evening
__1 Black __1 Metallic

Shoes
Closed Toe
__1 Black __1 Brown __1 Neutral

Open Toe
__1 Black __1 Brown __1 Neutral

Casual Sandals
__1 Black __1 Brown __1 Neutral

Boots
__1 Tall __1 Ankle __1 Neutral

Tennis Shoes
___1 White

Belts

Thin

__1 Black ___1 Brown __1 Metallic

Wide

__1 Black __1 Brown

Notes:

_____

_____

_____

_____

_____

_____

_____

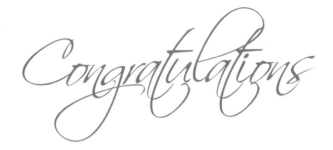

Congratulations

You're done! Doesn't it feel great? We are at the end of the program, but you are in the most amazing second half of your life. It is important for you to acknowledge your efforts and celebrate your success. You deserve it! Take a moment to congratulate yourself for the huge step you have just completed.

Thank you so much for trusting me to be your partner in helping you to develop your style over 40 from the inside out. It has truly been my pleasure to share some of the most personal and exciting experiences of my own journey of transformation with you, and help you facilitate yours. I trust that since you have completed the program, the insights and results you have gained will be long lasting and fulfilling . . . Enjoy!

Sybil

P.S. I'd love to hear your feedback about the program. Please, visit me at www.TheStyleConcierge.com. I have truly enjoyed building this program for you and look forward to hearing from you soon!